OCCUPATIONAL THERAPY
EVALUATION FOR
CHILDREN
A Pocket Guide

OCCUPATIONAL THERAPY EVALUATION FOR CHILDREN
A Pocket Guide

SHELLEY MULLIGAN
PhD, OTR/L

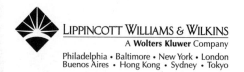

LIPPINCOTT WILLIAMS & WILKINS
A **Wolters Kluwer** Company

Philadelphia • Baltimore • New York • London
Buenos Aires • Hong Kong • Sydney • Tokyo

Senior Acquisitions Editor: Timothy L. Julet
Managing Editor: David Payne
Marketing Manager: Aimee Sirmon
Project Editor: Jennifer Ajello
Typesetter: Lippincott Williams & Wilkins
Printer: Malloy, Inc.

530 Walnut Street
Philadelphia, Pennsylvania 19106

351 West Camden Street
Baltimore, Maryland 21201-2436 USA

The publisher is not responsible (as a matter of product liability, negligence or otherwise) for any injury resulting from any material contained herein. This publication contains information relating to general principles of medical care that should not be construed as specific instructions for individual patients. Manufacturers' product information and package inserts should be reviewed for current information, including contraindications, dosages and precautions.

Printed in the United States of America

Library of Congress Cataloging-in-Publication Data
Mulligan, Shelley.
   Occupational therapy evaluation for children : a pocket guide / Shelley Mulligan.
      p. ; cm.
   Includes index.
   "Complement to the book titled "Occupational Therapy Evaluation for Adults" by Maureen Neistadt"--Pref.
   ISBN 0-7817-3163-1
   1. Occupational therapy for children--Handbooks, manuals, etc. 1. Neistadt, Maureen E. Occupational therapy evaluation for adults. II. Title.
   [DNLM: 1. Occupational Therapy--Child--Handbooks. WB 39 M959o 2003]
RJ53.O25M85 2003
615.8'515'083--dc21   2002043423

The publishers have made every effort to trace the copyright holders for borrowed material. If they have inadvertently overlooked any, they will be pleased to make the necessary arrangements at the first opportunity.

To purchase additional copies of this book, call our customer service department at **(800) 638-3030** or fax orders to **(301) 824-7390**. For other book services, including chapter reprints and large quantity sales, ask for the Special Sales department.

For all other calls originating outside of the United States, please call **(301) 714-2324**.

Visit Lippincott Williams & Wilkins on the Internet: http://www.lww.com. Lippincott Williams & Wilkins customer service representatives are available from 8:30 am to 6:00 pm, EST, Monday through Friday, for telephone access.

06 07
3 4 5 6 7 8 9 10

PREFACE

In working with children and their families, occupational therapists are concerned with performance in daily life, including play and school activities, and how their clients socially participate within their families and communities. The evaluation process is central to the services offered by occupational therapy. Evaluation focuses on uncovering what clients want and need to do and on identifying factors that support or act as barriers to their performance in daily activities. The occupational therapist's skilled observation and interview skills and ability to administer and interpret a variety of specific assessment tools and to synthesize data from multiple sources leads to a clear delineation of relevant problem areas. In pediatrics, evaluations of children provide the basis for the development of intervention plans and are valued as an integral part of more comprehensive, interdisciplinary developmental and functional evaluations of children.

This book is a complement to the book titled "Occupational Therapy Evaluation for Adults," by Maureen Neistadt. Its purpose is to provide occupational therapists, particularly novice practitioners and students, with a comprehensive and practical guide for conducting evaluations of children. It will serve well as a text for occupational therapy courses that cover content related to pediatric evaluation, assessment, and measurement. As a step-by-step guide, it could also be used as a procedures manual in laboratory courses. It is assumed that students and practitioners using this book have a background in normal and abnormal child development, occupational therapy theory and practice, and basic measurement principles. Given this background knowledge, this book was designed to include all of the necessary information to guide therapists through the evaluation process. The evaluation process described is consistent with the concepts included in the Occupational Therapy Practice Framework, adopted by the American Occupational Therapy Association (AOTA) (written by AOTA's Commission on Practice, 2002). This document was created to describe the domain that centers and grounds the occupational therapy profession and to outline the evaluation and intervention process. It was published in December 2002, and it is currently available from AOTA's Web site, www.aota.org.

As an occupational therapy clinician, instructor, and researcher, I am committed to the provision of quality occupational therapy services. In creating this resource, I have put together content that assists therapists and students in developing skills necessary to conduct evaluations reflecting a high standard of care. Evaluating children is a complex process. In addition to applying the technical aspects of interviewing, conducting observations, and administering and interpreting tests, therapists must perform these functions in ways that are comfortable for the child's caregivers and fun for the child. I value the extra time it takes to really get to know the children who are referred and to involve caregivers throughout the evaluation process. It is the initial interactions during evaluation activities that form the basis of trusting relationships.

Chapter 1 begins by identifying the main characteristics of the systems and settings within which occupational therapists work in pediatrics. System and setting factors, including legislation that supports and guides occupational therapy services in various medical and educational settings must be considered throughout the evaluation process. Chapter 2 includes the step-by-step process of evaluation. Background information on normal child development, with particular attention to the typical occupations and skills of children of different ages, is provided in Chapter 3 to help therapists select appropriate evaluation activities and interpret evaluation data.

I feel strongly that therapists need to become aware of the strengths and limitations of the evaluation techniques and tools they use. Chapter 4 covers issues related to standardized testing, including how to interpret test scores and factors to consider in selecting assessment tools, and provides detailed information on evaluating the psychometric properties of standardized tests. Chapter 5 covers nonstandardized evaluation techniques, including interviews and observations. Information gained from informal interviews and observations often provide the most valuable data, particularly for intervention planning. Therefore, ideas for conducting and documenting observations of children during play, school, and other functional activities performed in their natural contexts are emphasized. The content in Chapter 6 focuses on teaming and provides guidelines for conducting collaborative evaluations.

The content in Chapter 7 augments the material in Chapter 2 regarding the final two steps of the evaluation process: the interpretation and synthesis of evaluation data for intervention planning and the communication and documentation of evaluation results. Sample evaluation reports and intervention plans are included, as well as tips for writing intervention goals. Throughout the book, much of the content is presented in tables, boxes, and figures for quick and easy access to the information, and key terms are presented in bold face.

ACKNOWLEDGMENTS

The vision and many of the ideas for this book originated from Maureen Neistadt, who created the adult version of this book in 2000. She saw a need for a similar book for occupational therapists working with children. As a friend, colleague, and mentor, I thank her for the confidence she had in me to tackle this project on my own and for the many years she devoted to the profession, to her students, and to her patients. I hope that I was able to convey the importance of taking a gentle, sensitive, kind approach when evaluating children and their caregivers. It was the ease with which Maureen approached students and clients in this way that set her apart from others. One of the important lessons she would have wanted readers to gain from this book is to always place the client's needs before one's own.

I thank David Payne and Ulita Lushnycky at Lippincott Williams and Wilkins, who both functioned as managing editors during different phases of the book. David, your gentle persistence, your ability to attend to and manage details, and your words of encouragement helped me get this book to press.

Several of my family members and friends agreed to be photographed for the book. I thank you for generously giving of your time to do so and for being so photogenic, especially Scott, Eric, Jessie, KC, Lindsay, Enin, Sam, and Jake. Lisa Nugent and her crew from the photography department at the University of New Hampshire are extremely talented, and they coped well with having to chase little people around and amuse toddlers while they waited their turns.

I would also like to thank my husband Ted for his love, patience, and support. It was with his interest in my work, encouragement, assistance with all of the everyday tasks of life that a husband and wife raising three busy children need to do, and sense of humor that this book has come to completion.

REVIEWERS

Joanne Jackson Foss, MS, OTR
Department of Occupational Therapy
University of Florida
Gainesville, FL

Michele Biro, MS, OTR/L
Kennedy Child Study Center
New York, NY

Bonnie J. Hacker MHS, OTR/L
Occupational Therapist
Durham, NC

Tana L. Hadlock, MA, OTR
Occupational Therapy Department
University of Texas at El Paso
El Paso, TX

Anita W. Mitchell, MS, OTR, BCP
The University of Tennessee Health Science Center
Memphis, TN

Kathi L. Adams, MS, OTR/L
Division of Occupational Therapy
Shenandoah University
Winchester, VA

Rebecca Thomas, OTR
Pediatric Occupational Therapist
Memphis, TN

Elizabeth Werner DeGrace, PhD, OTR/L
Department of Rehabilitation Science
University of Oklahoma
Oklahoma City, OK

Cyndi Haynes, MEd, OTR/L
Occupational Therapy Program
Philadelphia University
Philadelphia, PA

JoKaren S. Werner, MA, OTR
Occupational Therapy Department
Newman University
Wichita, KS

CONTENTS

CHAPTER 4
STANDARDIZED ASSESSMENT TOOLS

CHAPTER 5
INTERVIEWS AND OBSERVATIONS

CHAPTER 6
WORKING AS A MEMBER OF A TEAM

CHAPTER 7
INTERVENTION PLANNING AND
DOCUMENTATION

APPENDICES

TABLES

CHAPTER 3

CHAPTER 4

BOXES

CHAPTER 6

CHAPTER 7

APPENDIX A

FIGURES

CHAPTER 4

CHAPTER 5

CHAPTER 6

CHAPTER 7

APPENDIX E

1

PEDIATRIC OCCUPATIONAL THERAPY EVALUATION ACROSS PRACTICE SETTINGS AND SYSTEMS

INTRODUCTION TO THE EVALUATION PROCESS

Occupational therapy evaluation is both a set of procedures and a thought process. Although the terms "evaluation" and "assessment" are often used interchangeably, in this book they will be distinguished, consistent with definitions provided by the American Occupational Therapy Association (AOTA) (Neistadt and Crepeau, 1998). Evaluation is the process of obtaining and interpreting data necessary for intervention, whereas assessment refers to using a specific "tool," such as a standardized test. The set of procedures involved in pediatric evaluation typically includes administering standardized and nonstandardized developmental, functional, and skill-specific assessments; interviewing; and conducting observations of children during age-appropriate activities and within various contexts and settings (Stewart, 2000).

The thought process in pediatric occupational therapy evaluation is similar to the process used by therapists in other practice areas. It involves a way of thinking about the information gathered and how it should be interpreted. This thought process also helps determine what information you, as the occupational therapist, still need to complete the evaluation and how you will go about getting this new information. The act of evaluating is a mental process whereby therapists constantly observe and interact with clients and their families to gain a clearer picture of client problems, strengths, and priorities and begin to hypothesize about possible intervention strategies. You will engage in the evaluation thought process during evaluation procedures and during all other interactions with the children with whom you are working. That is, occupational therapy practitioners are evaluating client problems, strengths, and progress during both evaluation and intervention sessions. The evaluation thought process is ongoing from the first through the last meeting with the client.

The process of occupational therapy evaluation described in this book is based on the new **Occupational Therapy Practice Framework** adopted by the AOTA (AOTA, 2002). Important pieces of this document related to evaluation are included in Appendix A.

One of the first decisions you will often need to make is whether an occupational therapy evaluation is warranted. Therefore, sometimes a **screening** is necessary. A screening involves gathering preliminary information for the sole purpose of determining whether an evaluation is necessary. Activities involved in a screening vary and may include conducting a telephone interview with a parent or referral source, conducting a classroom observation or examining some classroom work, reviewing medical or educational records, or administering a standardized assessment tool designed as a screening instrument.

The remainder of this chapter focuses on three areas that contribute significantly to the evaluation process in pediatrics and that provide some essential background information to prepare you for evaluating children and their families. First, the clinical reasoning process that guides your decision making throughout the evaluation process is discussed further. Second, the importance of the family is emphasized because in pediatrics both the child and the caregivers are considered your clients. The roles of family members throughout the evaluation process are discussed along with methods for examining family functioning. Third, characteristics of the most common practice settings and systems for pediatric occupational therapy are discussed. Although the underlying philosophy of occupational therapy, the principles of evaluation, and the importance of considering both the child and the family remain stable across practice settings, some characteristics of various practice settings are unique and affect how occupational therapy evaluations are carried out. The most common practice settings for pediatric occupational therapists include (1) early-intervention, community-based programs; (2) preschools and other school settings; (3) community mental health programs, residential programs, and outpatient clinics; and (4) inpatient hospital settings. The characteristics of these common practice settings and how they influence the occupational therapy evaluation process are presented.

CLINICAL REASONING

Clinical reasoning is a multifaceted, cognitive process used by occupational therapists to plan, direct, perform, and reflect on their client services (Schell, 1998). It is important that you use different types of clinical reasoning during the evaluation thought process (Neistadt, 1998). Table 1-1 defines the different types of clinical reasoning and provides examples of how each is used during occupational therapy evaluation and intervention. Your occupational therapy evaluations and interventions will be most effective when you use narrative reasoning first because understanding the client's life story (family and child priorities, concerns, lifestyle, medical history, etc.) will help you focus on what is most important. Narrative reasoning enables you to think about the child and family as unique, human individuals and not as a set of problems. Consequently, the evaluation sequence suggested in Chapter 2 is client centered and uses narrative reasoning throughout to ensure that the child's needs and priorities are being adequately addressed throughout the evaluation process.

Chapter 2 also suggests that you focus your procedural reasoning by using a **top-down approach** to evaluation (Stewart, 2000). With this approach, you start by gathering information about the child's needs, problems, and con-

TABLE 1-1 | TYPES OF CLINICAL REASONING USED DURING EVALUATION

Type of Clinical Reasoning	Definitions	Practitioner Actions	Contributions to the Evaluation Process
Narrative	Yields the child's occupational story, emphasizing his or her preferred activities, habits, roles, and family priorities. Also encompasses the client's and therapist's story together by identifying how the client and therapist will work together to build a meaningful future for the child and family.	Interview the child and family about routine activities, childrearing practices, activity preferences, school, and social history.	Focuses on family and child goals, increasing participation, and motivation; helps build the child's occupational profile.
Interactive	Yields an understanding of what the disease or disability means to the child and the family, i.e., the child's illness experience. Also encompasses interpersonal interactions between therapists and clients.	Therapeutic use of self; working collaboratively with children and families.	Enhances child motivation and participation and child and family satisfaction. Ensures that the intervention is fun and rewarding for the child.
Procedural	The process of defining clients' diagnosis-related problems with (1) their routine life activities, (2) the skills	Evaluation of procedures and administration of assessment tools, activity analysis, and use of activity	Identifies clients' OT problems and interventions appropriate for managing those problems.

	needed to perform those activities, and (3) the environments where those activities occur and then selecting appropriate interventions.	as a therapeutic modality.	
Pragmatic	Used to consider all of the practical issues that affect OT services: the intervention environment and system; the therapist's and team's values, knowledge, and abilities; client social and financial resources; and materials.	Knowledge and monitoring of reimbursement systems, knowledge of system policies and regulations, effects of the environment on clients, and knowledge of client resources.	Identifies intervention options with collaborative decision making to select the best intervention for the given situation or setting. Transition/discharge planning.
Ethical	Used to choose a morally defensible course of action with clients in the face of competing interests.	Ongoing attention to the client's goals and their relation to the goals of caregivers and providers. Following AOTA ethical standards.	Identifies ethical interventions for any given client. Evidence-based practice.
Conditional	Used to revise the intervention moment to moment to meet the client's needs. This revision is done in consideration of the client's current and possible future contexts.	Flexibility with respect to OT services in any particular session.	Better client participation. Highlights the importance of activity analysis to discover the therapeutic potential of all activities.

AOTA, American Occupational Therapy Association; OT, occupational therapy.

cerns regarding valued occupations and daily life activities. This information is then used to develop an **occupational profile** of the child (Occupational Therapy Practice Framework) (AOTA, 2002) (see Appendix A). An occupational profile describes the client's occupational history, patterns of daily living, interests, values, and needs. Developing an occupational profile involves identifying and then examining children's abilities to perform the activities that are part of their everyday lives, i.e., those activities that they value and that give meaning to their lives (e.g., play, school activities, interactions with family members, and self-help tasks). Information for developing a child's occupational profile is often obtained through interviews with caregivers, the child, and other family members. In addition, observations of children in action—performing their self-care skills, playing at a playground, interacting with their family members and peers, and engaging in school activities for school-aged children—are helpful in developing occupational profiles. Occupational profiles are essential for understanding child and family priorities, and these priorities guide the services that you as the occupational therapist ultimately offer.

The second step in the evaluation process is to generate and test hypotheses to determine factors that support or hinder the child's ability to engage successfully in their valued occupations. This second step has been termed an "analysis of occupational performance" (AOTA Practice Framework) and involves examining children's abilities to carry out their daily activities. Examination of child factors such as underlying motor, process, or interaction skills (sometimes referred to as performance components) and assessment of the demands of the activity and contextual factors are required to help identify why the child is experiencing difficulty. Hypotheses generated may then be explored further by administering formal assessment tools to examine specific child factors (motor, process, or interaction skills) identified as possible deficit areas. A table listing client factors is included in the Occupational Therapy Practice Framework (see Appendix A).

This top-down approach first helps you identify the functional performance problems of concern to the children and families referred to you and then assists you in identifying those component skills that seem problematic. One of the most important contributions of occupational therapy to client care in pediatrics is the identification of barriers that prevent a child from participating in his or her valued occupations and the subsequent implementation of strategies to remove the barriers. Focusing on the most relevant barriers, whether they are child component skills or environmental factors, allows the evaluation process to be more efficient. This efficiency is vital in today's health care and educational systems.

FAMILY PARTICIPATION IN THE EVALUATION PROCESS

The occupational therapy evaluation process in pediatrics is unique in that the child's family members, particularly the caregivers, are just as integral (if not more so in many cases) to the evaluation process as the child. Just like establishing rapport with your client (the child), establishing rapport and trust with the child's parents (also your clients) is essential for providing effective occupational therapy services. Most important, the child's caregivers, and their home environment, will always have a greater impact on the child's development and ultimate functional performance than you or any other professional involved on a temporary basis (Baloueff, 1998). Your recommendations will or will not be realized through the actions of family members. Therefore, the nature of the partnership you create with the family and your skills in empowering them to carry out their day-to-day caregiving responsibilities must be reflected throughout the evaluation and intervention process.

Specific guidelines and requirements for including parents and guardians in the evaluation and program planning process are included in legislation for providing early-intervention services and preschool and other school-based services (Individuals With Disabilities Education Act [IDEA], 1997, Parts B and C). Early-intervention services (for children younger than 3 years), which are described in more detail later herein, follow a family-centered model. In this model, caregivers are central team members who assist in developing all aspects of the services provided to their child. It is, however, important that you, as the occupational therapist, be sensitive to the concerns, needs, and priorities of family members regardless of your practice setting.

The typical, specific roles of caregivers or parents and other family members during the evaluation process include (1) interviewee or provider of information; (2) participant supporting and assisting the child and you, the evaluator; (3) participant examining aspects of family functioning and quality of interactions among family members, and (4) collaborator in the exchange of information (sharing and receiving) and in problem solving and decision making throughout the evaluation process.

As a provider of information, caregivers often give the child's medical history and may complete questionnaire-type assessment tools such as a sensory profile questionnaire, behavior rating scales, or functional evaluations. It is important to gain information from the perspective of family members regarding the child's strengths and weaknesses, likes and dislikes, and typical activities and environments. The concerns, priorities, hopes, and dreams for the child and for the family unit are vital pieces of information for developing the child's occupational profile and for determining important areas for further evaluation and intervention. The child's caregivers know their child best. Therefore, caregivers provide a wealth of information throughout the evaluation.

A second role is for caregivers and sometimes siblings to assist during the administration of evaluation activities, particularly for infants and young children who may not perform well with strangers. Infant assessments are often designed to have test items administered by caregivers. Depending on the purpose of the evaluation, it may be important to observe parent-child play behaviors, social play with siblings, and family members engaging in other daily activities.

Third, an understanding of family functioning and of the home environment is important in consideration of the influence of the family system on a child's development. Specially designed assessment tools of family functioning may be completed by family members, and informal observations of the home environment may be important, as well as evaluation activities designed to examine the typical interactions, roles, cultural influences, and habits of families.

Finally, client-centered practice means focusing on the needs and priorities expressed by your clients—the child and family members. Encouraging caregivers and older children to actively participate in the process of decision making for identifying other areas for further evaluation and to exchange information throughout the evaluation process assists in establishing rapport and in gathering important information about their values and their goals for intervention. It is crucial for you to listen to their ideas, concerns, and priorities as you begin the process of intervention planning together with the family.

SETTING AND SYSTEM CONSIDERATIONS IN PEDIATRIC EVALUATION

Early-Intervention, Family-Centered Services

Federal support for early-intervention services has been made a priority because current research indicates that early-intervention services are helpful in (1) promoting positive developmental and functional outcomes in children at risk for developmental problems and (2) preparing young children to be successful as they enter their school years. Part C of the IDEA (101-476, 1997) (see Appendix B) was developed to assist communities in implementing collaborative, multidisciplinary, interagency, early-intervention services for children with disabilities from birth through their second year and for their families. Services are typically provided in natural settings (most often the home) and follow a family-centered, medically oriented philosophy.

In early intervention, you will typically evaluate children and their families collaboratively with other professionals as a member of an interdisciplinary or transdisciplinary team (see Chapter 6). With a family-centered philosophy, the parents' concerns, strengths, and priorities must be accounted for throughout the evaluation process and during the development and implementation of the intervention program, which is called the individual family services plan (IFSP). Team evaluations must determine eligibility for services, which includes the following criteria: (1) established risk (children with a known disability such as Down's syndrome), (2) developmental delays, as measured by appropriate, standardized developmental assessment tools; and (3) at risk for developmental problems, which may include both environmental risk factors, such as having a single, teenaged mother, and biological risk factors, such having a low birth weight. Specific evaluation requirements under Part C of the IDEA are included in Table 1-2.

Family-centered service is based on several important principles. It is assumed that parents know their child best and want the best for him or her. All families are diverse and special, and family members contribute unique and important perspectives during the evaluation process and throughout intervention. Also, a family's stress management and coping skills can greatly affect the child's ability to function (King et al., 1998). In family-centered care, the professional collaborates with the family as a partner rather than being the "expert." Services are based on the family's strengths and are culturally sensitive and flexible (Prelock et al., 1999).

Parents have stated that the principles of family-centered care and interdisciplinary practices are most effective in meeting the challenges that they and their children with disabilities face and in supporting their lives in the contexts that are most meaningful: home and community (Prelock et al., 1999). An interdisciplinary team consists of professionals who provide services beyond their specific domain, overlapping roles and integrating knowledge to address the multifaceted needs of the family (Prelock et al., 1999). Family members tend to value professional cooperation and organization and to believe that a team of professionals who bring many different perspectives is best suited to meet the complex needs of their children with disabilities (Prelock, 1999). Chapter 6 provides more indepth information on conducting team evaluations.

Young children with mental health conditions and disorders such as nonorganic failure to thrive, autism, attachment disorders, and multisystem, regulatory disorders of

TABLE 1-2	INDIVIDUALS WITH DISABILITIES EDUCATION ACT PART C: INFANTS AND TODDLERS FROM BIRTH TO AGE 3 YEARS
Issue	**Description**
Eligibility	An infant or toddler younger than 3 years who needs early-intervention services because the individual is experiencing developmental delays in one or more of the areas of cognitive, physical, communication, social, or emotional development and in adaptive development or has a diagnosed physical or mental condition that has a high probability of resulting in developmental delay; may also include, at each state's discretion, at-risk infants and toddlers.
OT services	Supportive service to assist a child with a disability to benefit from special education. OT is a service provided by a qualified occupational therapist and includes (1) improving, developing, or restoring functions impaired or lost through illness, injury, or deprivation; (2) improving the ability to perform tasks for independent functioning if functions are impaired or lost; and (3) preventing, through early intervention, initial or further impairment or loss of function.
Evaluation policies	A statewide system shall provide (1) a multidisciplinary assessment of the unique strengths and needs of the infant or toddler and identification of services appropriate to meet such needs; (2) a family-directed assessment of the resources, priorities, and concerns of the family and identification of the supports and services necessary to enhance the family's capacity to meet the developmental needs of the infant or toddler; and (3) periodic review, including evaluation of the IFSP once a year and review of the plan at 6-month intervals (or more often where appropriate based on infant or toddler and family needs) and within a reasonable time after completion of the assessment.
Intervention programs	A written IFSP developed by a multidisciplinary team, including the parents. The IFSP must include the child's current levels of development; a family-directed assessment of resources and priorities, expected child outcomes, and the criteria, procedures, and timelines to determine the degree to which progress toward goals is being achieved; whether modifications or revisions of the outcome or services are necessary and a statement of specific intervention services, frequency, intensity; and payment arrangements, if necessary.

IFSP, individual family service plan; OT, occupational therapy.

infants and young childhood may also be addressed through early-intervention programs. Parental mental health conditions such as a history of substance abuse or depression may place young children at risk for developmental concerns, neglect, or abuse, and, therefore, such families may also be referred for evaluation and interventions by early-intervention teams.

Although most occupational therapy services for children from birth through the second year of life are provided through federally supported and governed family-centered, early-intervention programs, not all of our services for this age group are delivered under this system. Occupational therapy evaluations may also be conducted for this age group in hospitals and outpatient medical clinic settings, in privately funded community programs, and in mental health community and residential programs.

Educational Settings: Occupational Therapy as a Related Service

In the United States, evaluations for school-aged children are often mandated and to some degree are controlled by federal legislation. Congress has passed laws that include many different parts and sections. Some of the parts and sections are especially relevant for occupational therapy, whereas others are more relevant for administrators and others. Each law is labeled "PL" for "Public Law" and is given a number and a date when the bill was passed. Legislation of major concern to occupational therapists working with children in schools includes (1) the IDEA (PL 105-17) (IDEA, 1997), which is education legislation, and (2) Section 504 of the Vocational Rehabilitation Act of 1973, which, similar to the Americans With Disabilities Act, is human rights legislation.

Occupational therapy, as defined under Part B of the IDEA (1997) (see Appendix C), is a related service provided to students aged 3 to 21 years who are eligible for special education and who have been identified as having occupational therapy needs. Occupational therapists working in schools must follow the regulations set forth in the IDEA. In this setting, occupational therapy evaluations are conducted for any of the following reasons: (1) to determine a child's eligibility for services, (2) to determine the child's level of functioning (and progress) in any number of educationally relevant activities at various times, and (3) to assist in the development of student individual education programs (IEPs). Occupational therapists in schools work with children who have all types of physical, cognitive, behavioral, and social deficits.

School occupational therapists, whether they are placed in preschool programs or in elementary or high schools, work collaboratively with other education team members, such as general and special education teachers and speech pathologists, to design and carry out IEPs. As with early intervention, evaluations are often conducted collaboratively with other team members, and information about how team evaluations are conducted and the role of the occupational therapist in this process are discussed in detail in Chapter 6.

It is important to keep in mind that occupational therapy services in schools may address only those child factors and skill areas considered educationally relevant or that impact the child's ability to participate successfully in school activities (IDEA, 1997). For example, in the area of self-care or self-maintenance activities, occupational therapists may evaluate a student's level of independence in the lunchroom, his or her ability to use the bathroom at school, and his or her capacity to get dressed to go outside for recess or for gym class. Addressing the student's ability to use the bathtub at home or to organize a morning self-care routine independently before school may not be considered educationally relevant. Medically oriented interventions such as occupational therapy activities to increase range of motion after a hand injury or occupational therapy using sensory integration techniques in a clinic setting only (without application in the context of the educational setting) are often beneficial for certain children but may not be considered educationally relevant. Therefore, these interventions are carried out in medically oriented clinic settings and are rarely paid for by the educational system. However, it is not uncommon for school-aged children to receive services from more than one setting or system.

In addition to considering educational relevance, the IDEA stipulates that all special education services that include occupational therapy must be provided within the least restrictive environment in which the child's services can be effectively provided. This requirement has played an important role in gaining overwhelming support during the past decade for inclusive education. This means that as much as possible special education services are provided in the child's regular classroom environment and in the context of typical classroom activities. It is therefore essential that you, as the occupational therapist, specifically evaluate how children perform in their school environments and include classroom observations of the child as part of an evaluation. Occupational therapy evaluations under the IDEA should also consider aspects of the child's curriculum and daily routine at school because this information helps determine the environmental demands and expectations placed on a child.

As noted previously, the IDEA, Part B, mandates special education services for children aged 3 to 21 years, which encompasses programs for children at the extreme age ranges: preschool services and prevocational, vocational programs or other day programming for young adults with disabilities. Services for preschool children are typically carried out in special education or integrated preschool programs housed in public elementary schools, or services are provided in community preschool settings. Students aged 18 to 21 years may continue in regular high school settings with special education and related services, or they may be supported by school personnel in community programs and settings. In addition, programs outside a school district, from for-profit and nonprofit agencies, are sometimes contracted by school districts to provide services for children who reside in their districts if the home school district does not have the resources or if program options are believed to be appropriate for a particular student.

School-based evaluations take place at designated times. First, an initial evaluation to determine eligibility for services may occur any time a child is approaching 3 years or older and is suspected of having difficulties in any area of development. Standardized assessment tools are often required because they are more likely to provide diagnostic information and they provide standardized scores of functional performance. These assessment data are helpful for making eligibility decisions and for educational coding (children eligible for special education must fit under at least one educational diagnostic code). All children receiving special education services must have a formal, comprehensive evaluation at 6 years of age, and then every 3 years thereafter. In addition, yearly evaluations are necessary specifically for the development of IEPs. Specific influences of federal regulations governing school-based evaluations are summarized in Table 1-3, and relevant policies and definitions included in the IDEA are given in Appendices B and C.

In addition to receiving special education services through the regulations set forth in the IDEA, school-based occupational therapy services for children may be provided through civil rights legislation. A "504 plan," which is based on part of the revised Rehabilitation Act of 1973, ensures that students with disabilities are given equal access to activities (such as school activities) in public and private organizations and that reasonable accommodations are made to allow students to access such activities (see Appendix D). You may be asked to conduct occupational therapy evaluations to determine whether students can access their desired activities and, if not, to determine what accommodations would be necessary to allow access. Evaluations related to Section 504 must include contextual evaluations (i.e., assessment of the student performing the activities they need to do at school in the natural settings), as well as evaluations of performance areas within those contexts. Specific characteristics of occupational therapy services under Section 504 are summarized in Table 1-4, and relevant policies and definitions included in Section 504 are given in Appendix D.

Outpatient Community Programs, Residential Settings, and Outpatient Clinics

As part of a children's hospital or a rehabilitation hospital, multidisciplinary outpatient clinics are sometimes available for children with specific chronic conditions, such as

TABLE 1-3	INDIVIDUALS WITH DISABILITIES EDUCATION ACT PART B: PRESCHOOL AND SCHOOL CHILDREN AGED 3 TO 21 YEARS
Issue	**Description**
Eligibility	A child aged 3–21 years identified and coded with a disability, which means that a child was evaluated as having one or more of the following conditions: mental retardation; hearing impairment, including deafness; speech or language impairment; visual impairment, including blindness; serious emotional disturbance; an orthopedic impairment; autism; traumatic brain injury; another health impairment; a specific learning disability; deaf-blindness; or multiple disabilities and who, by reason thereof, needs special education and related services.
OT services	OT is a supportive service required to assist a child with a disability to benefit from special education provided by a qualified occupational therapist and includes (1) improving, developing, or restoring functions impaired or lost through illness, injury, or deprivation; (2) improving the ability to perform tasks for independent functioning if functions are impaired or lost; and (3) preventing, through early intervention, initial or further impairment or loss of function. Services may be provided indirectly through consultation, supervision, and monitoring of others or directly in groups or individual sessions.
Evaluation policies	In general, a state or local educational agency shall conduct a full and individual initial evaluation before the initial provision of special education and related services to a child with a disability. Such initial evaluation shall determine whether the child has a disability and shall identify the educational needs of the child. A local educational agency shall ensure that reevaluation of each child with a disability is conducted if conditions warrant reevaluation, if the child's parent or teacher requests reevaluation, or at least once every 3 years. The local educational agency shall provide notice to the parents describing any evaluation procedures the agency proposes to conduct. In conducting the evaluation, the local educational agency shall (1) use a variety of assessment tools and strategies to gather relevant functional and developmental information; (2) include information provided by the parent that assists in determining whether the child has a disability; (3) include information helpful in determining the content of the child's IEP, including information related to enabling the child to be involved in the general

TABLE 1-3	INDIVIDUALS WITH DISABILITIES EDUCATION ACT PART B: PRESCHOOL AND SCHOOL CHILDREN AGED 3 TO 21 YEARS *(Continued)*
Issue	**Description**
Evaluation policies	curriculum or, for preschool children, to participate in appropriate activities; (4) not use any single procedure as the sole criterion for determining whether a child has a disability or in determining an appropriate educational program for the child; and (5) use technically sound instruments that may assess the relative contribution of cognitive and behavioral factors in addition to physical or developmental factors.
Intervention programs	A written IEP developed by an educational team that includes the classroom teacher, the parent, and the child when appropriate. The IEP must include the student's current level of educational performance, annual goals and short term measurable objectives, the special education and related services that will be provided and the extent and location of the services, dates for initiation of and anticipated length of services, evaluation procedures and schedules to obtain data to determine whether the objectives are being met, and transition services for children 12 years and older.

IEP, individual education program; OT, occupational therapy.

cerebral palsy, juvenile rheumatoid arthritis, or muscular dystrophies. Some clinics are also designed to address specialized problems, such as dysphagia (feeding and swallowing disorders) and assistive technology needs (including wheelchair evaluations, computer needs, and augmentative communication). The primary role of occupational therapists in these settings is often one of evaluation and consultation around programming needs. Direct services, for example, on a weekly basis, may also be provided on a short-term basis. Sometimes therapists who work in these clinics act as consultants for other therapists who work more regularly with the children, such as school-based occupational therapists.

Community clinics in pediatrics are also available to provide specialty interventions such as sensory integration interventions or programming for children and adolescents with psychosocial, emotional disabilities or problems.

TABLE 1-4	SCHOOL-BASED SERVICES UNDER SECTION 504 OF THE VOCATIONAL REHABILITATION ACT
Issue	**Description**
Eligibility	An individual with a disability who requires reasonable accommodations to participate in or have equal access to major life activities (school activities and environments) provided by both the private and public sectors.
OT services	May be a support or primary service required to evaluate and determine the needs of students with disabilities for accommodations to enable them to participate fully in school activities; may involve development of a 504 service plan and implementation and monitoring of the 504 plan.
Evaluation policies	Written documentation is needed that describes the student's disability, the impact the disability has on the student's ability to perform school activities, and the accommodations needed to allow the student to fully participate in all school activities.
Intervention programs	A written 504 plan stating the accommodations that are necessary and how they will be provided.

OT, occupational therapy.

Often, such clinics, programs, or therapists who work in specialized areas are contracted by school agencies or early-intervention programs to provide specialized services that they cannot offer in their districts. The percentage of occupational therapists working specifically in child mental health is relatively small (approximately 10% of practicing therapists, AOTA member survey, 1990), although we have a wealth of skills to provide services in the mental health area. Outpatient mental health services are provided through several different types of settings, such as freestanding clinics, community mental health centers, and hospital outpatient programs. Funding sources include Medicaid, federal grants, health insurance, and private pay. In 1992, the Comprehensive Community Mental Health Services for Children and Their Families was authorized by Congress. This federal program provides funding to state agencies to organize and provide mental health services for children and families.

Residential treatment centers are another type of setting available for children with significant mental health and behavioral concerns. Although these centers do not typically address acute problems, residential programs provide more structure, restrictions, and safety than do day programs. Lengths of stay in residential treatment programs vary tremendously from weeks to several years, with the goal being to prepare children and adolescents for successful return to the community and their families. Education programs are most often provided on-site, although sometimes children may attend other private or public schools. In residential settings, occupational therapists may provide related services as a part of a child's IEP (through IDEA legislation) or may provide evaluations and interventions through the medical and mental health systems.

Private practice is another option for occupational therapists. Therapists may establish their own practice and provide services for children and their families on an outpatient basis. They may also contract their services to early-intervention programs, school programs, or other community programs. Reimbursement for occupational therapy services provided for children in private pediatric clinics may be obtained through contractual agreements with agencies such as school systems or from health insurance, private pay, and Medicaid. Each of these payer sources has its own regulations and policies with respect to reimbursement guidelines and requirements. Specifically related to evaluations, some health insurance companies, for example, may require you to be a member of their network to bill for services, some may require previous authorization, and some may reimburse for certain kinds of diagnostic codes and evaluation procedures only. The most common diagnostic codes and evaluation codes used for reimbursement from health insurance companies, including health maintenance organizations, for occupational therapy evaluations are listed in Table 1-5. Therefore, before conducting occupational therapy evaluations in outpatient clinic settings, it is essential that you familiarize yourself with the billing and reimbursement policies and are prepared to follow any procedures that are required by the agency that is being billed for the services. These codes are updated frequently, so you will need to keep informed on an ongoing basis.

TABLE 1-5	COMMON *ICD-9* AND *CPT* CODES FOR BILLING PEDIATRIC OT SERVICES[a]

ICD-9 Codes (Diagnosis)	*CPT* Codes (OT Services)
299.0 Autism	96110 Developmental testing
315.4 Developmental coordination disorder	96115 Neurobehavioral status examination
314 Attention-deficit hyperactivity disorder	97110 Therapeutic exercise
315.8 Delay in development (specified)	97112 Neuromuscular reeducation
315.9 Delay in development (unspecified)	97530 Therapeutic activities
348.3 Encephalopathy	97535 Self-care/ADLs
343.9 Cerebral palsy	97533 Sensory integrative techniques
349.9 Unspecified disorder of the nervous system	
758.0 Down's syndrome	
768.9 Intracranial hemorrhage	
312.8 Conduct disorder	
313.81 Oppositional defiant disorder	
309.21 Separation anxiety disorder	

[a]This is not a complete listing; codes are periodically updated.

ADLs, activities of daily living; *CPT, Current Procedural Terminology; ICD-9, International Classification of Diseases, Ninth Revision;* OT, occupational therapy.

Inpatient Hospital Services

Occupational therapists commonly provide services in a variety of hospital settings and programs, including neonatal intensive care units and other special care nurseries, acute care, mental health programs, and rehabilitation services for children. They typically work as a members of multidisciplinary teams. This means that occupational therapists perform their own individual occupational therapy evaluations and collaborate with other team members on a regular or informal basis to share information and to develop comprehensive and efficient programs (Sparling, 1980).

Hospital programs have their own set of policies and procedures to be followed with respect to occupational therapy evaluation. For example, there may be time stipulations for how quickly evaluations must be completed and available in the medical chart from the time a referral is received. Specific guidelines and procedures may be provided for documenting an evaluation, and sometimes specific evaluation forms must be completed as part of the evaluation process. Occupational therapy services in hospital-based pediatric programs are almost always initiated through physician orders. Multiple sources of data, including review of the medical records, use of standardized and nonstandardized tests, and functional observations and interviews, are typically used in the evaluation process. The main purposes of evaluations are to determine levels of functioning, to establish programming needs, and, in some cases, to obtain diagnostic information.

It is your responsibility as the therapist to be aware of and to follow the policies and procedures in the hospital setting in which you work. Pediatric hospital services are typically funded by health insurance carriers, including private insurance companies, health maintenance organizations, and Medicaid. Preauthorization for occupational therapy evaluation services may be necessary, and if services are recommended by occupational therapy, evidence must be provided in the evaluation regarding the medical necessity of the intervention and the predicted functional outcomes or rehabilitation potential.

Historically, children who required rehabilitation services, for example, because of head trauma or a spinal cord injury, stayed in the hospital for months and even years in some extreme cases (Dungeon, 2000). Today, school-based programs and other community outpatient centers and home-based programs and supports have taken over much of the rehabilitative roles of therapists in hospital-based programs. Therefore, hospital programs today emphasize the more acute phases of illness or injury or the evaluation and treatment of children with more rare and complex medical conditions.

Children referred for your services in hospital settings may therefore be medically fragile because of the acute nature of their medical conditions. Care must be taken during the evaluation to monitor vital signs such as heart and respiratory rates, to follow precautions to prevent the spread of infection, and to follow any other necessary precautions. Before beginning your evaluation with a hospitalized child, it is recommended that you speak to the child's nurse to obtain up-to-date information on the child's medical status and medical precautionary procedures that need to be followed.

SUMMARY

This chapter introduced occupational therapy evaluation as a client-centered, top-down process. The process begins with the development of an occupational profile of a child, and then moves to evaluation activities to uncover the factors that hinder or promote a child's ability to successfully engage in daily, valued occupations. The relationship between clinical reasoning and evaluation was presented, and AOTA's Practice Framework was introduced as the basis for the evaluation process described in this book. Family members were identified as our clients, along with the children referred for our services, and the important roles of family members throughout the pediatric occupational therapy evaluation process were explained. Finally, the various practice settings and systems in which pediatric occupational therapists typically work were described, including early-intervention, family-centered community programs; educational settings; outpatient community mental health programs; residential settings and outpatient clinics; and inpatient hospital programs. Specific setting and system characteristics, such as special education laws and issues regarding health insurance reimbursement, that directly impact the evaluation process were discussed.

The next chapter provides a guiding framework to help you go through the process of evaluation in a step-by-step manner, with detailed descriptions of the actions to be addressed at each step.

References

American Occupational Therapy Association (2002). Occupational Therapy Practice Framework: Domain and process. *American Journal of Occupational Therapy, 56,* 609–639.

Baloueff, O. (1998). Introduction to the pediatric population. In M.E. Neistadt & E.B. Crepeau (Eds.), *Willard & Spackman's occupational therapy* (9th ed., pp. 569–575). Philadelphia, PA: Lippincott Williams & Wilkins.

Dungeon. B. (2001). Pediatric rehabilitation. In J. Case-Smith (Ed.), *Occupational therapy for children* (4th ed, pp. 843–863).

Individuals With Disabilities Education Act (IDEA) Amendments of 1997 (Pub L No.105–17), USC 1400.

King, G., Law, M., King, S., & Rosenbaum P. (1998). Parents' and service providers' perceptions of the family-centeredness of children's rehabilitation services. *Physical and Occupational Therapy in Pediatrics, 18*(1), 21–37.

Neistadt, M. (1998). Teaching clinical reasoning as a thinking frame. *American Journal of Occupational Therapy, 52,* (3), 221–229.

Neistadt, M. & Crepeau, E.B. (1998). Glossary. In M.E. Neistadt & E.B. Crepeau (Eds.), *Willard & Spackman's occupational therapy* (9th ed., pp. 866–873). Philadelphia, PA: Lippincott Williams & Wilkins.

Prelock, P.A., Beatson, J., Contompasis, S.H. & Bishop, K.K. (1999). A model for family-centered interdisciplinary practice in the community. *Topics in Language Disorders, 19*(3), 36–51.

Schell, B. (1998). Clinical reasoning: The basis of practice. In M.E. Neistadt & E.B. Crepeau (Eds.), *Willard & Spackman's occupational therapy* (9th ed., pp. 90–100). Philadelphia, PA: Lippincott Williams & Wilkins..

Sparling, J.W. (1980). The transdisciplinary approach with the developmentally delayed child. *Physical and Occupational Therapy in Pediatrics, 1*(2), 3–16.

Stewart, K. B. (2001). Purposes, processes and methods of evaluation. In J. Case-Smith (Ed.), *Occupational therapy for children* (4th ed, pp. 190–213).

2
A GUIDE TO EVALUATION

INTRODUCTION

Evaluation is the process of gathering and interpreting information about children and their families. Evaluations are performed for many reasons, such as to identify a diagnosis, to evaluate progress, or for research and program evaluation purposes. This chapter focuses on the evaluation process for determining a child's eligibility and need for further occupational therapy services and for program planning purposes. According to the **Occupational Therapy Practice Framework of the American Occupational Therapy Association** (AOTA, 2002) (see Appendix A), the evaluation process consists of two main parts: (1) development of an **occupational profile** and (2) **analysis of occupational performance.** The occupational profile describes the individual and his or her occupations. Analysis of occupational performance involves examining relevant performance skills (motor, process, and communication) and client factors (body function and structures) that support occupational performance. In addition to client factors, analysis of occupational performance involves examination of specific activity demands and of the contexts in which the activities and occupations are typically performed.

It is important that you are aware of the language adopted by the World Health Organization to define various levels of human functioning because this was the language that the AOTA incorporated into its Practice Framework. This language provides a useful, consistent system for understanding and communicating on national and international levels issues of importance related to the functional competencies of individuals with disabilities. The purpose of the **International Classification of Impairments, Activities, and Participation** (ICIDH-2) (World Health Organization, 1998) is to classify human functioning at the level of the body, the whole person, and the person within their social and physical environmental contexts. The ICIDH-2's consideration of "participation" and "activities" largely reflects the AOTA's recommendation that you first develop the child's occupational profile and that environmental factors and activity demands need to be considered in the evaluation of one's ability to participate in meaningful activity. Evaluation of "body functions" and "body structure," as defined by the ICIDH-2, comprises the client factors that may be considered important for further evaluation during the analysis of occupational performance. Specific definitions for the main concepts of the ICIDH-2, and the relationships among the ICIDH-2 terminology, the AOTA's uniform terminology (AOTA, 1994), and the terminology used in the AOTA's Practice Framework are included in Appendix E. Updates on the ICIDH-2's new language can be found at www.who.int/icidh.

Figure 2-1 depicts the steps that you will go through in conducting your evaluations after a referral is received. The rest of the material in this chapter provides detailed information regarding each of the steps.

STEPS IN THE EVALUATION PROCESS

STEP 1   Gather Relevant Background Information

The amount and type of available background information will vary tremendously from setting to setting. For example, in hospital settings you will have the medical record to review, and in school settings you may have a special education file to review if the student had received special education in the past. The amount of information provided as a part of the referral will also vary. For example, you may receive a referral in a hospital setting that just states,

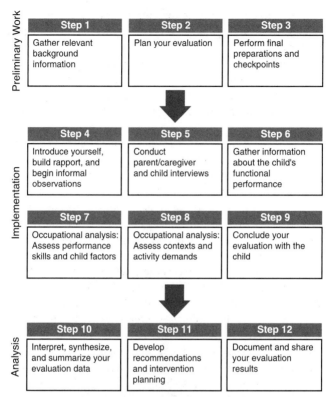

Figure 2-1 The 12-step occupational therapy evaluation process.

"occupational therapy evaluation and treatment," with only the name, sex, age, diagnosis, and room number. In a school setting, you may receive a referral that states, "occupational therapy evaluation and treatment of fine motor difficulties; child is currently receiving special education for a learning disability." If the nature of the child's problems or reasons for the referral are unclear, then it is important for you to obtain clarification from the referring source. At the very least, you should feel knowledgeable about the reasons for the referral and should be aware of the main presenting problems that triggered the referral. This clarification often requires a telephone interview with the referral source (a parent, teacher, or physician). Obtaining this background information may also be considered part of a screening to determine whether the referral for an occupational therapy evaluation is appropriate and necessary.

A specific diagnosis or educational coding provides some initial information about common problems associated with the diagnosis that may need to be addressed or about precautions that may need to be observed during your evaluation. Medical records are also helpful in identifying evaluations and assessment tools that have been used and about the timing of their use. Information about a young child's ability to separate from their caregivers or to perform for strangers, about a child's likes and dislikes, or about a child's ability to sit at a table and follow directions (required for administering many standardized assessment tools) is very useful for planning your evaluation activities.

Common sources of **preevaluation information** include (1) medical records, (2) school records, (3) reports from other professionals (medical or educational personnel) who have seen the child, (4) interviews with parents or other caregivers, and (5) interviews with the referral source, teacher, or physician. Gathering information about the child's diagnosis, presenting problems, and reasons for referral is essential before seeing the child. More detailed information regarding the child's medical history, birth history, timing of developmental milestones (such as sitting up and walking), and involvement with any past or current medical or special education services and programs is also important to gather at some point during the evaluation process. Interviews to gather such evaluation data may be conducted before seeing the child, during the evaluation session, or after evaluation of the child. Chapter 5 provides more detailed information about conducting client interviews.

STEP 2   Plan Your Evaluation

Planning your evaluation involves scheduling a time to see the child and selecting the assessment tools, materials, and activities that you will use during your evaluation. It is important for you to schedule a time that will be comfortable for the child and for other individuals who are affected by or contribute to the evaluation. These "others" may include nursing staff, teachers, and, of course, parents. It is important to be sensitive to the time of day, child/family schedules, etc., when finding a time that is convenient for all parties involved and that will help elicit the most meaningful and reliable evaluation information. There may also be legal or institutional guidelines that dictate how soon your occupational therapy evaluation should take place after a referral is received.

Selecting the most useful assessment activities, tools, and materials requires a great deal of clinical reasoning and is one of the more difficult parts of the evaluation process because you need to consider so many factors (e.g., child and family characteristics, the purpose of the evaluation, your skills, and the environment) when creating your evaluation plan. Three types of evaluation procedures are available: (1) administration of standardized assessment tools; (2) nonstandardized but formal procedures, observations, and interviews; and (3) informal observations, including naturalistic observations. For most evaluations, you will probably use all three of these procedures. Detailed information about evaluating, selecting, and using standardized, norm-referenced, and criterion-referenced assessment tools is provided in Chapter 4. Chapter 5 covers nonstandardized assessment procedures in more depth, including interviewing and conducting formal and informal clinical and naturalistic observations.

Information on normal development is also important to consider in the evaluation planning process (see Chapter 3). This information helps you (1) form appropriate and relevant interview questions, (2) select appropriate toys and activities for the evaluation, (3) gain insight into effective ways to approach children of various ages and developmental levels, and (4) interpret the evaluation data.

You will consider many different factors as you engage in the clinical reasoning process throughout the planning and preparation steps of your evaluation (see Table 1-2). Examples of evaluation plans that may be used with children of various ages and with certain diagnosis

TABLE 2-1	SAMPLE EVALUATION PLANS FOR INPATIENT HOSPITAL SETTINGS	

Setting/Age/ Diagnosis	Standardized Assessments	Nonstandardized Procedures
Neonatal intensive care unit/31 weeks' gestation/prematurity, bronchopulmonary dysplasia	NAPFI (Dubowitz and Dubowitz, 1981)	Medical history, including maternal prenatal history; infant's birth history; current medical status (equipment, feeding, medications, homeostasis, precautions); interview nursing; observe state regulation, including level of arousal, auditory and visual orientation, cry, and consolability; feeding, muscle tone, posture, movement patterns, and selected reflexes; interview parents; observe infant-parent interactions
Rehabilitation unit/5 years old/ traumatic brain injury; alert	Wee-FIM (Hamilton and Granger, 1991); MVPT-R (Colarussi and Hammill, 1995); Ranchos LOCF-r (Hagen, 1998)	Interview nursing, parents, and child; gather information about child's interests, activities, and school program; observe IADLs; neuromuscular function (tone, movement patterns, strength, balance, coordination, fine and gross motor skills); observe process and communication skills during IADLs and play, including global and specific mental functions and behavior

or referring problems in different practice settings are included in Tables 2-1 to 2-4. However, it is important for you to understand that every child referred to you comes with a unique combination of individual and contextual characteristics that will affect your decisions as you plan your evaluation activities. Sometimes you will need to conduct your evaluation activities in more than one session, and often in more than one setting. A perfect set of evaluation activities that will work for all chil-

TABLE 2-1	SAMPLE EVALUATION PLANS FOR INPATIENT HOSPITAL SETTINGS (*Continued*)

Setting/Age/ Diagnosis	Standardized Assessments	Nonstandardized Procedures
Rehabilitation unit/17-years-old/ C5-6 spinal cord injury	COPM (Law et al., 1994)	Interview client and family members; formally test sensory functions; test functional movement, range of motion, and manual muscle strength; observe client performance of IADLs; evaluate for high and low technology, including the need for a power wheelchair and other adaptive devices to assist with IADLs, and for participation in desired occupations
Mental health unit/14 years old/anorexia nervosa	Adolescent Role Assessment (Black, 1976); AMPS (Fisher, 1994)	Interview child and parents; gain information about the child's self-esteem and self-control; expressive person drawing; time management and activity log; observations during social and leisure activities and during mealtime

AMPS, Assessment of Motor and Process Skills; COPM, Canadian Occupational Performance Measure; IADLs, instrumental activities of daily living; MVPT, Motor Free Visual Perception Test; NAPFI, Neurological Assessment of the Preterm and Full-term Infant; Ranchos LOCF-r, Ranchos Levels of Cognitive Function–Revised; Wee-FIM, Functional Independence Measure for Children.

dren with a specific diagnosis or set of challenges does not exist. Therefore, careful planning is crucial for all of your evaluations.

STEP 3 Perform Final Preparations and Checkpoints

Some **last minute preparations** or considerations are necessary before your evaluation, and these preparations will

TABLE 2-2	SAMPLE EVALUATION PLANS FOR OUTPATIENT CLINIC SETTINGS

Setting/Age/ Diagnosis	Standardized Assessments	Nonstandardized Procedures
Clinic specializing in SI disorders/ 7 years old/DCD	SIPT (Ayres, 1989); Sensory Profile (Dunn, 1999); TVMS-R (Gardner, 1995)	Caregiver, teacher, and child interviews emphasizing their concerns with the child's occupational performance, the child's interests, and parent/child priorities; observations of fine and gross motor skills during play and school-related activities; formal observations of postural control, muscle tone, balance, and coordination
Child development clinic/4 years old/ Down's syndrome	PDMS-2 (Folio and Fewell, 2000); Vineland ABS (Sparrow et al., 1984); Sensory Profile (Dunn, 1999)	Caregiver interview; observations of the child's motor, process, and communication skills during IADLS, including feeding and dressing, and during play
Cerebral palsy clinic/ 16 years old/spastic quadriplegia, seizure disorder, MR (mental retardation)	COPM (Law et al., 1994); Person-Environment Fit Scale (Coulton, 1979)	Caregiver and teacher interviews; review of relevant medical records and current programs; classroom observations; assessment of motor skills through formal clinical observations of functional mobility, joint range of motion, muscle strength, sitting posture, transfers, upper limb coordination, and functional use; assessment of process and communication skills through observations of relevant functional IADLs (grooming and feeding); assess need for low and high technology related to seating, computer use, communication, and other devices to assist with IADLs and other valued activities

TABLE 2-2	SAMPLE EVALUATION PLANS FOR OUTPATIENT CLINIC SETTINGS (*Continued*)

Setting/Age/ Diagnosis	Standardized Assessments	Nonstandardized Procedures
Community mental health program/ 15 years old/ substance abuse	Adolescent Role Assessment (Black, 1976); Piers-Harris Children's Self-Concept Scale, Piers (1984)	Parent and child interviews; assess process and communication skills during structured group activities and during other relevant school-related, vocational, homemaking, and leisure activities

COPM, Canadian Occupational Performance Measure; DCD, developmental coordination disorder; PDMS-2, Peabody Developmental Motor Scales–2; SI, sensory integration; SIPT, Sensory Integration and Praxis Tests; TVMS-R, Test of Visual-Motor Skills–Revised; Vineland ABS, Vineland Adaptive Behavior Scales.

vary depending on your setting and specific situation. In all cases, you will need to gather assessment materials and forms. In a clinic setting, you may need to prepare the testing environment and set up testing materials. If your client is hospitalized, you should check with nursing staff, read recent notes in the medical chart to make sure that the child can be seen, and read any signs posted in the client's environment regarding medical precautions or care procedures. If you are doing the evaluation in the home, then it's best to call ahead to let the parents know that you are on your way. Finally, you need to clear your head and be ready to focus on the child and others involved in the evaluation, such as the parent or caregiver. Your keen, **informal observations** will probably be the most powerful and useful evaluation data. With your attention focused, you will truly be able to be there with the client during the evaluation.

STEP 4 Introduce Yourself, Build Rapport, and Begin Informal Observations

As you begin your evaluation, your first goal is to **establish rapport** with your clients (usually the child and a

TABLE 2-3	SAMPLE EVALUATION PLANS FOR EARLY INTERVENTION AND PRESCHOOL SETTINGS

Setting/Age/ Diagnosis	Standardized Assessments	Nonstandardized Procedures
Early intervention/ 9 months old/fetal alcohol syndrome	BSID-II (Bayley, 1993); TSFI (DeGangi and Greenspan, 1989); HOME-r (Caldwell and Bradley, 1984)	Caregiver interview; observations of caregiver and infant interactions and social play; observations of the infant's motor, process, and communication skills during play and during relevant IADLs, such as feeding
Early intervention/ 2.5 years old/ PDD-NOS	PDMS-2 (Folio and Fewell, 2000); KPPS-r (Knox, 1997); HELP (Furuno et al., 1984)	Caregiver interview; observations of caregiver and infant interactions and social play; observations of the infant's motor, process, and communication skills during play and relevant IADLs, such as feeding
Preschool/4 years old/cerebral palsy– spastic hemiplegia	PEDI (Haley et al., 1992); Classroom Observation Guide (Griswold, 1994)	Parent and teacher interviews; observations, including activity in the classroom and on the playground; assessment of neuromuscular factors, including tone, muscle strength, functional range of motion, balance, and motor coordination; bilateral hand use; observations of play skills, fine and gross motor skills
Preschool/5 years old/developmental delay	SFA (Coster et al., 1998); Miller Assessment for Preschoolers (Miller, 1988)	Parent and teacher interviews; observation of the child engaged in classroom and playground activities; assessment of sensory and motor factors, including tone, muscle strength, balance, and motor coordination; bilateral hand use; observations of play skills, fine and gross motor skills

BSID-II, Bayley Scales of Infant Development II; HELP, The Hawaii Early Learning Profile; HOME-r, Home Observation for the Measurement of the Environment–Revised; IADLs, instrumental activities of daily living; KPPS-r, Knox Preschool Play Scale–Revised; PDD-NOS, pervasive developmental disorder–not otherwise specified; PDMS-2, Peabody Developmental Motor Scales–2; PEDI, Pediatric Evaluation of Disability Inventory; SFA, School Function Assessment; TSFI, Test of Sensory Function in Infants.

TABLE 2-4	SAMPLE EVALUATION PLANS FOR ELEMENTARY, MIDDLE, AND HIGH SCHOOL SETTINGS

Setting/Age/ Disability	Standardized Assessments	Nonstandardized Procedures
Fourth grade/ 9 years old/learning and attention disorders	BOTMP (Bruininks, 1978); ETCH (Amundson, 1995); SFA (Coster et al., 1998)	Child, parent, and teacher interviews; sensory processing history; classroom observations; review of classroom written and other work; clinical observations of sensory motor functions, including postural tone, movement patterns, balance, strength, and coordination
Sixth grade/ 11 years old/ cerebral palsy, spastic diplegia, poor handwriting	School AMPS (Fisher and Bryze, 1997); TVMS-R (Gardner, 1995); TVPS (non-motor) (Gardner, 1997)	Child, parent, and teacher interviews; observations in school environments, with particular attention to functional mobility and written work; clinical observations of sensory motor functions, including postural tone, movement patterns, balance, strength and coordination
Eleventh grade/ 17 years old/ spinal muscular atrophy, type II	COPM (Law et al., 1994)	Child, parent, and teacher interviews, including a discussion of transition plans; observations in school environments and during participation in IADLs, school-related activities, and other activities of interest; evaluation of technology needs; indepth evaluation of feeding

(continued)

parent; in a school environment, this may be the teacher and child), and it is essential that you make them feel comfortable and that you are respectful. Some actions on your part that will help you accomplish this are as follows:

TABLE 2-4	SAMPLE EVALUATION PLANS FOR ELEMENTARY, MIDDLE, AND HIGH SCHOOL SETTINGS *(Continued)*

Setting/Age/Diagnosis	Standardized Assessments	Nonstandardized Procedures
Ninth grade/15 years old/moderate mental retardation and behavioral problems	School AMPS (Fisher and Bryze, 1997); Sensory Profile, adolescent/adult version (Brown and Dunn, 2002)	Child, parent, and teacher interviews; observations in school environments during school-related activities and during child's participation in relevant IADLS and vocational and leisure activities

BOTMP, Bruininks-Oseretsky Test of Motor Proficiency; COPM, Canadian Occupational Performance Measure; ETCH, Evaluation Tool of Children's Handwriting; IADLs, instrumental activities of daily living; School AMPS, School Version of the Assessment of Motor and Process Skills; SFA, School Function Assessment; TVMS-R, Test of Visual-Motor Skills–Revised; TVPS-R, Test of Visual Perceptual Skills (Non-Motor)–Revised.

- always knocking before entering the client's space (home, hospital room, or classroom)
- introducing yourself and explaining the purpose of your visit to both the child and the parent using language appropriate to the child's developmental level
- asking how the client would like to be addressed and not addressing adults by their first name unless given permission to do so
- collaborating with the parent or teacher to determine the extent of their participation and presence in the evaluation process
- interacting or playing with the child in fun ways that make him or her feel successful and relaxed

From the moment you enter the child's space or environment (e.g., home or classroom), take note of any specific characteristics that may have the potential to enhance or hinder the child's performance. For example, are spaces cluttered or do they allow children to move freely? What materials, toys, and activities are accessible and available? Begin to make informal observations of the child's behavior, such as attention, affect, language use, activity level, and reactions to you as a stranger. Also, be attentive to the needs of the child and parent(s), read body language, and adjust your behavior to maximize their comfort level with the evaluation process. Sometimes this means joining in and doing whatever the child was already doing before initiating the new activities that you have planned.

STEP 5   Conduct Parent/Caregiver and Child Interviews

Informal interviews with the child (children older than 3 or 4 years) and his or her parent(s) are helpful to gain information about the child's interests, strengths, and challenges and will help you uncover **child and family priorities**. They also give you an opportunity to establish rapport with your clients and for you to explain what you hope to accomplish throughout the evaluation process. Interviews are also useful for gathering initial information about the child's functional performance, which is emphasized in Step 6 of the evaluation process. The interview should be more like a conversation than like a question-and-answer period. You should ask questions that are largely based on what your client has just told you. Using this method of asking questions ensures that you have **listened carefully** to the client. Your questions should be open ended so that they require more than a simple yes or no answer and should not be biased in the way that they are worded. Specific techniques and example interview questions are provided in Chapter 5, and some standardized assessment tools that follow structured interview formats are included in Chapter 4.

Because it is almost always necessary that you interview the caregivers as well as older children, the timing of the parent/caregiver interviews can be tricky. For example, parents may not want to talk to you about their child's difficulties with the child present, but the child requires supervision; or the parents may not be able to relax and focus during an interview because they are distracted by their child. It is important, therefore, that you are thoughtful in your evaluation planning about when and where these interviews take place. Some suggestions for managing challenging situations are as follows:

- interview the child during the context of a play situation and while you are making informal observations
- consider a telephone interview with the parent either before the evaluation or shortly after (before is better because you may gain insights into important factors or areas to focus on with the child during the evaluation)
- set up the child with favorite toys near you and the parent(s) either at the end or the beginning of the evaluation session while you speak with the parent(s)
- talk with the parents while you work with the child (this works sometimes with very young infants); however, it is not highly recommended because it is difficult to establish a relationship with the child when you are talking with the caregiver, and it is very difficult (if not impossible) to gather information from the parent and the child simultaneously
- explain to the parent ahead of time that you would like time to talk to them about their main concerns and priorities, and have them problem solve with you about how this can take place; sometimes another adult can be present at the evaluation to watch the child while the interview takes place

STEP 6   Gather Information About the Child's Functional Performance

When using a **top-down approach** to evaluation, you begin by gathering information about the child's ability to perform functional skills and to perform successfully in roles and activities that are meaningful to him or her. **Areas of occupation** that you may want to address are listed in the AOTA's Practice Framework (see Appendix A). Areas of occupation include activities of daily living (ADLs), such as self-care activities; instrumental ADLs, which for children may include activities related to care of pets, homemaking and chores, money management, and school and work activities; and activities related to play and leisure. Information about abilities to perform in areas of occupation may already be gathered from your interviews with the child and caregivers. Information about the child's functional performance can also be acquired effectively through informal observations, particularly naturalistic observations. For example, if a child has feeding difficulties, observing him or her eat a meal or a snack is helpful. If the child has difficulty following a classroom routine, then it would be important for you to do a classroom observation, particularly at a time when the child must make transitions from one activity to the next. If a mother is concerned about her infant's social interactions while they play, then it would be important for you to observe them playing together.

While making observations of a child's performance, you should be answering several questions: How does the child perform the task? How much and what type of assistance does the child require? What kinds of compensations is the child making? What specific performance components or child factors (e.g., sensory, motor, cognitive, and emotional) seem to be hindering the child's performance? What task demands or environmental factors are affecting the child's ability to perform the activity?

Common terminology used by occupational therapists to **describe the amount of assistance** required or the level of independence of a child ranges from being totally dependent, requiring varying degrees and types of assistance, to being fully independent. This terminology is described in detail in Box 2-1 (Rogers and Holm, 1998; Trombly and Quintana, 1989).

Various standardized assessment tools are also available for gathering evaluation data regarding a child's functional abilities (see Table 2-5). The most common **pediatric functional assessment tools** include the School Function Assessment (Coster et al., 1998), the Vineland Adaptive Behavior Scales (Sparrow et al., 1984), the Pediatric Evaluation Disability Inventory (Haley et al., 1992), the Assessment of Motor and Process Skills (Fisher, 1999; and school version, Fisher and Bryze, 1997), and the Canadian Occupational Performance Measure, third edition, by Law

BOX 2-1	TERMINOLOGY USED TO DESCRIBE LEVELS OF ASSISTANCE

Dependent: Child requires assistance with >75% of the task or is unable to perform any aspects of the task.

Maximal assist: Child requires assistance with 50%–75% of the task.

Moderate assist: Child requires assistance with 25%–50% of the task

Minimal assist: Child requires assistance with up to 25% of the task.

With verbal cues: Child is able to perform the task when given verbal cues.

Supervision: Child is able to perform the task independently but requires supervision for safety or when occasional assistance is needed.

Task set up: Child can perform the task independently when the necessary environment or materials are set up.

Independent with assistive devices: Child is independent with appropriate assistive devices or technology.

Totally independent: Child is independent with all aspects of the task without the use of adaptive equipment or techniques.

Adapted from Rogers JC, Holm MB. Evaluation of activities of daily living (ADL) and home management. In: Neistadt ME, Crepeau EB, eds. Willard & Spackman's Occupational Therapy. 9th Ed. Philadelphia: Lippincott Williams & Wilkins, 1998:185–208; and Trombly CA, Quintana LA. Activities of daily living. In: Trombly CA, ed. Occupational Therapy for Physical Dysfunction. 3rd Ed. Baltimore: Williams & Wilkins, 1989:386-410.

et al. (1994). Using standardized assessment tools is particularly helpful when it is important for you to obtain objective data on the functional outcomes or gains you aim to achieve. Standardized functional assessment tools also help direct your attention to the functional areas giving the child the most difficulty and, in some cases, those functional skills most valued by the child or the caregivers.

By the end of this step, you should have ample evaluation data to formulate an occupational profile of the child you are evaluating. In addition, you should be ready to develop hypotheses about factors that hinder or facilitate the child's ability to engage successfully in his or her valued occupations.

TABLE 2-5 PEDIATRIC FUNCTIONAL ASSESSMENT TOOLS USED BY OCCUPATIONAL THERAPISTS

Assessment Tool	Author(s)	Age Range	Main Purpose(s)
Pediatric Evaluation of Disability Inventory	Haley et al., 1992	6 months to 7.5 years	Assesses self-care, functional mobility, and social functioning through structured interview and/or observation; considers level of caregiver assistance and use of adapted devices
School Function Assessment	Coster et al., 1998	Kindergarten through sixth grade	Criterion-referenced tool for evaluating child performance, level of participation, and need for assistance in school activities, including both physical and cognitive/behavioral tasks
Assessment of Motor Processing Skills	Fisher, 1994	Versions for adults, adolescents, and young children, and a new school version	The child is asked to perform 5–6 tasks from a list of 56 calibrated ADL tasks. The tool measures process and motor skills as they relate to task performance, provides information about how the child is performing in a given context, and is used to predict performance in ADL areas
Vineland Adaptive Behavior Scales	Sparrow et al., 1984	Birth through 18 years	Measures communication, daily living skills, socialization, and motor skills; uses a behavior rating scale that is completed through a structured parent interview

(continued)

TABLE 2-5 | PEDIATRIC FUNCTIONAL ASSESSMENT TOOLS USED BY OCCUPATIONAL THERAPISTS *(Continued)*

Assessment Tool	Author(s)	Age Range	Main Purpose(s)
Canadian Occupational Performance Measure	Law et al., 1994	Can be completed by the parent on the child's behalf (for younger children)	Measures the child's (or the parents') perception of the child's performance and satisfaction in areas of self-care, leisure, and productivity; helpful for prioritizing intervention goals and for measuring functional outcomes
Self-Assessment of Occupational Functioning	Henry et al., 1999	Child version and adolescent-adult version	Self-report measure to be completed during a structured interview; based on the Model of Human Occupation; addresses strengths and weaknesses related to volition, habituation, performance, and environment
Functional Independence Measure for Children	Hamilton and Granger, 1991	Child version is for those aged 6 months to 6 years	Universal tool designed to measure rehabilitation outcomes related to functional skills, including self-care, mobility, sphincter control, communication, and social cognition
Klein-Bell Activities of Daily Living Scale	Klein and Bell, 1982	All ages (except infants and toddlers)	Rating scale that measures six areas of function: dressing, elimination, mobility, bathing and grooming, eating, and emergency telephone communication

ADLs, activities of daily living.

STEP 7 Occupational Analysis: Assess Performance Skills and Child Factors

There is no specific order for evaluating **performance skills** or **client factors**, although it is important that you consider the child's physical endurance, attention span, emotional well-being, etc., when making decisions about which areas to evaluate first. The performance skills that need to be evaluated vary among children and are based on hypotheses that you develop to help explain "why" a child is having difficulty performing his or her daily occupations. Also, the referral source may have stated specifically some areas for you to pay attention to in your evaluation, such as fine motor skills. The performance areas included in the AOTA's Practice Framework (see Appendix A) include (1) **motor skills**, such as posture, mobility, strength, endurance, and coordination; (2) **process skills**, such as mental energy, general knowledge, and organizational abilities; and (3) **communication skills**, including social relationships. Performance skills refer to behavior, i.e., to what an individual "does," whereas client factors refer to what a client "has."

The AOTA's Practice Framework has in many ways replaced what was previously termed the AOTA's uniform terminology (AOTA, 1994). Performance skills and child factors were referred to as performance areas and performance components in the AOTA's uniform terminology (AOTA, 1994). In deciding which child factors and performance skills require further evaluation, it may be helpful to examine the old uniform technology included in Appendix E as well as the areas and factors included in the Practice Framework (Appendix A). For the sake of organization, and to be consistent with the AOTA's Practice Framework, which was adopted by the profession in May 2002, specific evaluation procedures for the analysis of occupational performance are presented as they relate to the examination of motor, process, and communication skills. Procedures for evaluating specific client factors (body functions and structures) that support or contribute to one's ability to engage in the various performance skill areas are also presented.

Evaluation of Motor Skills

It is important to observe the child's ability to perform age-appropriate, meaningful fine, gross, visual-motor, and oral-motor skills in the context of play or leisure activities, self-care activities, preschool and school activities, and work activities (for older children only) (see Chapter 3). Several standardized assessment tools can be also administered to evaluate these areas (see Chapter 4) in children of various ages. Standardized and nonstandardized procedures for evaluating these components are summarized Tables 2-6, 2-7, and 2-8. Client factors contributing to one's ability to perform motor skills include bodily functions and structures related to sensory, neuromuscular, and movement functions. Therefore, more specific evaluation procedures related to each of these areas are presented in this section, under the general area of motor skills.

Evaluation of gross motor skills. In the gross motor area, it is important to evaluate the quality of movement and means of mobility for all children through caregiver interviews and observations of gross motor skills in the context that the child is using the skills. A young child's first steps, typically achieved between 10 and 15 months of age, is viewed as a major gross motor milestone and provides exciting new opportunities for the child to explore his or her environment and gain some independence. For preschool children, gross motor play includes competencies and safety negotiating playground climbers, slides, and swings and mastering the pedaling of the tricycle. Functionally, they need to learn to negotiate around obstacles in their home and preschool environments, climb stairs, balance when getting dressed, and keep up with the rest of the family on outings once they are no longer pushed in a stroller. Between 4 and 6 years of age, children learn many specific gross motor skills that further enhance their social play with others, such as swimming, skating, riding a bike, and playing soccer. In the elementary years, participation in sports activities, physical education, and unstructured gross motor play such as roller blading or ball play are important occupations. When evaluating children with significant movement disorders, specific areas to examine include their means of and level of independence

TABLE 2-6 PROCEDURES FOR EVALUATING GROSS MOTOR SKILLS AND PRAXIS

Specific Skill Area	Nonstandardized Procedures	Standardized Assessments
Gross motor skills	Observe and document the child's ability to perform age-appropriate gross motor skills (walking, running, jumping, climbing, hopping, skipping, playing on playground equipment, and playing ball; also see Chapter 3); during play and the performance of functional tasks such as dressing, reaching for and carrying objects, transfers, and negotiating around obstacles and over uneven ground, observe for indicators of balance, strength and endurance, agility and range of movement, coordination, and bilateral integration; ask the child or caregivers about the child's ability to ride a bike, swim, perform in physical education class, etc., and about participation and interest in sports activities	MAI (Chandler et al., 1980); PDMS-2 (Folio and Fewell, 2000); BOTMP (Bruininks, 1978); AIMS (Piper and Darrah, 1994); TIME (Miller and Roid, 1994); GMFM (Russell et al., 1993)
Motor planning or praxis	Observe and document the child's ability to perform novel motor tasks, to play with objects in different ways, to be creative with play, and to maneuver through obstacle courses; observe the child perform motor sequences or patterns following verbal directions and then in response to demonstration (imitation of postures games like Simon Says); note the child's ability to perform multistep functional tasks, such as simple meal preparation, playing sports games, dressing, watering plants, and building with construction toys	SIPT (Ayres, 1989); imitation of postures test items, such as those on the MAP (Miller, 1988)

AIMS, Alberta Infant Motor Scale; BOTMP, Bruininks-Oseretsky Test of Motor Proficiency; GMFM, Gross Motor Function Measure; MAI, Movement Assessment of Infants; MAP, Miller Assessment for Preschoolers; PDMS-2, Peabody Developmental Motor Scales–2; SIPT, Sensory Integration and Praxis Tests; TIME, Toddler and Infant Motor Evaluation.

TABLE 2-7 PROCEDURES FOR EVALUATING FINE MOTOR AND VISUAL-MOTOR SKILLS

Specific Skill Area	Nonstandardized Procedures	Standardized Assessments
Fine motor skills	Observe and document the child's ability to perform age-appropriate fine motor skills (such as reaching, grasping, and releasing objects; pencil skills; stacking 1-inch blocks; stringing beads; using scissors; lacing and doing up clothing fasteners; opening packages; self-feeding; and using a computer [see Chapter 3]); note the child's grasp patterns, dexterity, and in-hand manipulation skills, bilateral hand use, hand preference, and postural control and sensory factors influencing fine motor function	PDMS-2 (Folio and Fewell, 2000); BOTMP (Bruininks, 1978); Erhardt Developmental Prehension Assessment (Erhardt, 1994); Quality of Upper Extremity Skills Test (DeMatteo et al., 1993)
Visual-motor skills	Observe the child's ability to perform age-appropriate visual-motor activities, such as shape sorters; puzzles of varying difficulty; scissors use; pencil and paper tasks, including coloring, tracing, design copy, and handwriting; and ability to manipulate the computer mouse and play computer games	Test of Visual-Motor Skills-Revised (Gardner, 1995); Test of Visual-Motor Integration (Beery, 1997)

BOTMP, Bruininks-Oseretsky Test of Motor Proficiency; PDMS-2, Peabody Developmental Motor Scales-2.

TABLE 2-8	PROCEDURES FOR THE EVALUATION OF ORAL-MOTOR SKILLS

Specific Area or Skill	Nonstandardized Procedures
Oral-motor structures	Examine the oral structures, including lips, jaw, tongue, teeth, gums, and soft and hard palate
Oral-motor control, swallowing, and reflexes	Evaluate sucking, rooting, and tonic bite reflexes; note oral-motor movements during feeding, including chewing ability, lip closure on a spoon and cup, tongue movements, jaw control, initiation of the swallow reflex, and signs of aspirations; note ability to safely manage different food textures; note articulation difficulties
Oral praxis	Note the child's ability to imitate various mouth and tongue movements and movement sequences
Oral-motor sensitivity	Observe the child's response to touch inside and outside the mouth; ask about the child's food taste and texture preferences
Feeding history	Parents (and older child) should be questioned regarding the child's diet, body weight, and nutritional concerns; food preferences; and ability to tolerate and manage various food textures and consistencies

Adapted from Logemann JA. Evaluation and treatment of swallowing disorders. San Diego: College Hill Press, 1983; Morris SE, Klein MD. Pre-feeding Skills. Tucson: Therapy Skill Builders, 1987.

with mobility and their ability to access the environments that are important to them in their everyday life. In addition, it is important to determine whether they have opportunities to experience and participate in desired sports and other gross motor leisure pursuits, even if modifications are necessary. The roles of occupational therapists often overlap with those of physical therapists in the evaluation of gross motor skills. Therefore, it is important to be aware of the other services a child may be receiving in this area to avoid duplication of services.

Evaluation of fine motor performance and visual-motor skills. Occupational therapy evaluations tend to emphasize fine motor skill performance more than gross motor performance, probably because of the greater impact hand function has on one's ability to complete functional skills. Fine motor skills are used to perform most self-help skills, such as feeding, dressing, and grooming. School activities such as handwriting, computer use, and arts and crafts and homemaking tasks such as cooking, putting belongings away, and washing the car depend heavily on one's ability to use his or her hands. Therefore, making fine motor observations while a child performs some of these functional activities are helpful for determining how fine motor skills are impacting the child's ability to successfully perform the types of activities he or she need to do everyday. Standardized testing will assist you in determining the aspects of fine motor performance or upper extremity functions that are most problematic (e.g., dexterity, visual-motor integration, and hand strength) and also will provide you with a measure of how different a child's performance is from that of other children of the same or a similar age.

Visual-motor integration refers to how the eyes and hands work together, and tests of visual-motor skills often include items such as tracing and design copy (see Bruininks, 1978). Children with handwriting concerns often perform poorly on tests of visual-motor skill. Administering tests of nonmotor visual perception and of fine motor dexterity and coordination will assist in determining whether visual-motor concerns are related more to difficulties in the area of visual perception or to the motor component. Clinical observations and some standardized tests used to measure visual-motor skills and fine motor skills are included in Table 2-7.

Motor planning. Motor planning or praxis involves both a cognitive component (ideation, planning, and sequencing) and a motor component (the physical execution of the motor behavior or task). Children with motor planning problems often appear clumsy. They may be slow to position themselves correctly for motor play and slow to initiate and learn new play activities. They may find it more challenging than other children to play with novel toys, and they may have trouble adapting to changes in routine or engaging successfully in new play situations. Children with motor planning problems often seem to lack creativity in their play. To evaluate motor planning abilities, observations of how a child engages in novel activities are important. Motor imitation of simple and gradually more complex body postures and motor sequences can also be conducted. There are also standardized tests, such as the Sensory Integration and Praxis Tests (Ayres, 1989), that measure areas of praxis (see Table 2-6). This particular test is ideal in that it breaks down praxis into many different types so that more specific information about the kinds of praxis problems a child may have can be determined.

Evaluation of oral-motor skills. The evaluation of oral-motor skills, particularly as they relate to feeding abilities, falls within the realm of occupational therapy, although you will often collaborate with speech pathologists in this area. An understanding of the anatomy of the mouth and pharynx and of the normal process of swallowing is essential for therapists working in the areas of feeding and oral-motor development (Morris and Klein, 1987). To protect you and the child you touch, wearing gloves is considered best practice when conducting an oral-motor/feeding evaluation because it involves contact with a mucous membrane.

Dysphagia is defined as difficulty in swallowing. Swallowing, which generally takes less than 2 seconds, includes a voluntary component called the oral phase and two involuntary components called the pharyngeal and esophageal phases (Logemann, 1983). The oral phase involves breaking up food placed in the mouth into a small bolus in preparation for swallowing and includes chewing and moving the food to the back of the tongue, which initiates the swallowing reflex. The pharyngeal phase is initiated with the swallow reflex and involves the following three events: (1) the soft palate elevates and the posterior pharyngeal wall constricts to close the nasal cavity; (2) the larynx elevates and the epiglottis folds downward to cover the open airway(the vocal cords also contract to protect the airway), and the bolus moves through the pharynx; and (3) the bolus moves past the closed airway and the cricopharyngeus muscle relaxes and opens to allow the bolus to pass into the esophagus. During the esophageal phase, the bolus passes through the esophagus to the stomach via peristalsis (Logemann, 1983).

Because feeding and swallowing is a life-threatening activity, it is essential that the parents or caregivers of the child be involved in the evaluation of feeding issues, including the oral-motor evaluation. A comprehensive oral-motor evaluation should include assessment of oral structures, swallowing abilities, oral sensitivity, oral-motor reflexes, and oral-motor movements and control, including the strength of the muscles around the face, mouth, neck and trunk, and tongue movements. Postural control factors such as muscle tone, trunk stability, and sitting posture should also be assessed because these factors influence oral-motor control.

Specific abilities related to feeding, including lip closure and chewing, should be assessed, ideally, in context (i.e., during the child's typical mealtime or snack time). In addition, caregivers (and the child when applicable) should be questioned regarding the child's diet, any body weight and nutritional concerns, food preferences, and ability to tolerate and manage various food textures and consistencies. Specific standardized and nonstandardized procedures for evaluation of oral-motor function are presented in Table 2-8. If it is determined that a child is experiencing swallowing difficulties and is at risk for aspiration, further evaluation of swallowing abilities via videofluoroscopy or modified barium swallow should be considered (Zerilli et al., 1990). If a videofluoroscopy has already been done, then the results of the evaluation need to be reviewed as part of your oral-motor evaluation.

Client factors related to sensory functions. An evaluation of sensory processing assesses the child's ability to take in, modulate, and process information from the sensory systems. A quick sensory screen should include tests for (or parent questions about) vision and hearing. Depending on the referral questions, other sensory systems that may need to be addressed include the tactile, proprioceptive, and vestibular systems. Various sensory history questionnaires are available that can assist you in gathering and organizing information from the child's parents or caregivers during an interview. Occupational therapy evaluations should also determine how identified sensory deficits, such as hearing or vision loss, impact an individual's ability to carry out his or her daily occupations. More thorough analysis of sensory processing can be accomplished by administering a standardized assessment tool, such as the Sensory Profile (Dunn, 1999), the Sensory Rating Scale (Provost and Oetter, 1995), the Sensory Integration and Praxis Tests (Ayres, 1989), or the Sensory Assessment (Cooper et al., 1993) (see Chapter 4). Some assessment tools are designed to measure the functioning of specific sensory systems. Techniques for evaluating each sensory system are presented in the following sections, including a selection of the most common tools used by occupational therapists for evaluating specific areas of sensory processing.

Visual and auditory processing Vision, the dominant sense used by humans to interact effectively in their environments, is critical to consider in the evaluation process. It is first important to ask caregivers if their child has a history of visual problems or if the child has had a vision evaluation. Reports from professionals who specialize in the evaluation and treatment of disorders related to vision and visual perception, such as an optometrist, an ophthalmologist, and a psychologist, may be helpful. Many aspects of vision assessment are outside the realm and expertise of occupational therapists, but some aspects of visual processing and visual perception can be directly evaluated by occupational therapists. In addition to understanding how children use vision to complete functional activities, screening for visual problems should always be part of the evaluation process, and procedures for doing so are included in Table 2-9.

Many standardized tests have been designed to evaluate nonmotor visual perceptual skills (e.g., form constancy, visual memory, visual and figure ground discrimination, visual closure, and spatial relations), such as the Test of Visual Perceptual Skills–Revised (Gardner, 1997) and the Motor Free Visual Perception Test–Revised (Colarussi and Hammill, 1995). Portions of other standardized tests, such as the Sensory Integration and Praxis Tests (Ayres, 1989) and the Miller Assessment for Preschoolers (Miller, 1988), also have some nonmotor visual perceptual test items (see Chapter 4). Psychologists often evaluate this area as well, and it is important to review assessment data from psychol-

TABLE 2-9	PROCEDURES FOR VISUAL SCREENING AND EVALUATION

Specific Area or Skill	Nonstandardized Procedures
Visual acuity	Ask the caregivers for the date of the child's last visual examination and if they have any concerns about their child's vision; observe the child's ability to visually track, localize, and focus on objects
Visual tracking and oculomotor control	Ask the child to follow your finger or an interesting object as you move slowly across the visual fields from left to right, straight up and down, and diagonally; watch specifically for smooth eye pursuits, ability to separate eye movements from head movements, saccadic movements, accuracy, and ability to cross the midline smoothly
Functional vision	Observe the child during tasks that require vision, such as puzzles, identification of objects and pictures, reading, sorting colors and shapes, locating items on a book page and in the environment, copying from the blackboard, computer use/play, ability to move through a space with obstacles, and finding objects in a busy background (such as locating items in a refrigerator or an eraser in a junk drawer)
Sensitivity to visual stimuli	Ask parents how the child responds to bright lights or sunlight; note how distractible the child is to visual stimuli in the environment

ogy reports when applicable. Clinical observations of visual perceptual skills can be conducted by watching a child engage in carefully selected play activities or functional tasks, such as creating block and pegboard designs, playing with Legos, drawing and writing, dressing activities, playing computer games, looking for hidden pictures in a confusing background, playing ball, and doing puzzles.

Oculomotor skills, including ocular fixation, visual tracking, and scanning abilities, can also be evaluated by occupational therapists. It is important to note that the vestibular system plays a role in the voluntary control of eye movements by controlling eye movements in response to head movement and assisting with one's orientation in space. For example, vestibular-ocular pathways help the eyes remain focused on an object while the head and body move. Clinical observations for evaluating oculomotor skills are included in Table 2-9. Standardized vision assessments that may be used include the Sensorimotor Performance Analysis (Richter and Montgomery, 1991), which measures visual tracking, visual avoidance, visual processing, and eye-hand coordination; the Erhardt Developmental Vision Assessment (Erhardt, 1989), which measures reflexive and voluntary eye movements; and the Pediatric Clinical Vision Screening for Occupational Therapists (Scheiman, 1991), which screens for accommodation, binocular vision, and ocular mobility.

When screening for auditory processing problems, note the child's ability to respond to simple and more complex verbal directions (without the use of visual cues). Note whether young children turn toward your voice or other noisy objects, such as a bell or squeaky toy. Inquire whether the child has had a formal hearing examination by an audiologist or physician screening. Reponses to auditory information can also be examined by asking caregivers or teachers how their children respond to verbal directions and loud noises and how distractible they are in noisy environments.

Somatosensory (tactile) processing The evaluation of somatosensory processing (response to touch input) includes assessing the discriminative system (perceiving and locating light touch and deep pressure touch and two-point discrimination) and the protective system (sharp versus dull touch, perceiving hot and cold, and testing for tactile hyperresponsiveness or hyporesponsiveness). Tactile receptors are found throughout the skin and generally are activated through touch input, including pain, pressure, and temperature. A complete evaluation of somatosensory functions may be warranted for children with neurologic diagnoses such as spinal cord injury, peripheral nerve damage, or head injury (see Table 2-10). More subtle problems with somatosensory processing may be identified in children with sensory integration prob-

TABLE 2-10 | PROCEDURES FOR THE EVALUATION OF SOMATOSENSORY (TACTILE) FUNCTIONS

Specific Area	Nonstandardized Procedures	Standardized Tests
Modulation of tactile stimulation	Observe the child's response during activities heavily loaded with tactile stimulation (sensory tables, finger paint, Play Dough); note the child's response to your physical handling; interview the child and/or parent regarding tolerance for touch (cuddling), grooming activities (e.g., bathing, brushing hair and teeth), clothing of various textiles, and food textures or other activities heavily loaded with tactile stimulation; ask if the child is aware when getting bumps and bruises	Sensory Profile (Dunn, 1999); Touch Inventory for School-Aged Children (Brasic-Royeen and Fortune, 1990)
Primary somatic functions: light touch, pain, temperature Consider the child's age in determining whether this testing is appropriate	Generally, apply stimulus proximal to distal on the dorsal and ventral surfaces of the arms (affected and nonaffected sides), randomly dispersed, and ask the child to point to where he or she was touched; with the child's vision occluded, light touch can be applied with the therapist's fingertip or a cotton swab; the child is then asked to locate where he or she was touched; pain stimulus can be applied with a safety pin using one sharp and one blunt end, and the child indicates whether the touch	

	was sharp or dull; to evaluate temperature, fill one test tube, capped with hot tap water and another with cold water; randomly place the tubes in contact with the skin for about 1 sec and ask the child whether the stimulus was hot or cold	Portions of the MAP (Miller, 1988); SIPT (Ayres, 1989)
Tactile discrimination	With the child's vision occluded, touch the child lightly on the hands or arms with your finger and see whether the child can identify where you touched him or her; determine whether the child can identify tiny objects (coins, paper clips, marbles, various-shaped blocks) in his or her hands when vision is occluded; observe fine motor dexterity and in-hand manipulation of small objects, with and without vision	

MAP, Miller Assessment for Preschoolers; SIPT, Sensory Integration and Praxis Tests lems. For example, poor tactile discrimination is thought to be associated with the development of body scheme and motor planning abilities and is believed to contribute to the development of fine motor skill (Brasic-Royeen and Lane, 1991). Children with tactile defensiveness (hypersensitivity to touch input) tend to avoid activities heavily loaded with tactile stimuli, such as grooming tasks, playing with art materials, wearing certain fabrics, and may avoid contact with others or feel stressed when with other children. These more subtle problems with tactile processing can be evaluated through standardized self-report or caregiver questionnaires as well as through clinical observations of children involved in activities heavily loaded with tactile stimuli. Specific procedures for evaluating somatosensory processing are included in Table 2-10.

Vestibular and proprioceptive processing The vestibular system includes neural receptors that are located in the semicircular canal, the utricle, and the saccule of the inner ear. This system is stimulated by movement of the head and is influenced by gravity. Vestibular functioning plays an important role in awareness of body position and movement in space and in postural control, which includes muscle tone, equilibrium and balance, and stabilizing the eyes in space during head movements (Fisher, 1991). Evaluation of vestibular processing should therefore include assessment of postural control factors, including righting, equilibrium, protective reactions, muscle tone, and balance skills (see Chapter 3 for a description of normal development of these reactions and other neuromotor functions).

The evaluation of postural control factors depends on the age of the child. In infants and young children, as well as older children with significant motor impairments (such as those with cerebral palsy), the focus is on whether they have achieved appropriate developmental motor milestones, the development of antigravity postures, the development of postural reactions, and integration of primitive reflex patterns. In older children (those ambulating well), your evaluation will involve assessing the child's postural control and proficiency during gross motor play and functional skills that require balance, such as riding a bike, going up and down stairs, playing hopscotch, walking on a balance beam, and getting dressed.

Proprioceptive processing refers to the functioning of specialized receptors located in the muscles and joints, and stimulated through active movement. Proprioception gives us information about the spatial orientation of our body, the rate and timing of our movements, the amount of muscle force being exerted, and how fast and how much a muscle is being stretched (Matthews, 1988; Fisher, 1991). Proprioception plays an important role in the development of body awareness and motor planning and in the accuracy of motor movements (Fisher, 1991). Because it is difficult to separate the contributions of the vestibular system from those of the proprioceptive system during motor performance, our clinical occupational therapy evaluation of these systems often occurs simultaneously.

In addition to examining postural control factors related to vestibular and proprioceptive processing, it is also important to evaluate the child's response to or modulation of vestibular and proprioceptive sensory stimuli. Children may be overly sensitive to certain types of movement activities and may crave others. For example, some children may fear heights and avoid climbing on playground equipment, whereas others may crave spinning and be constantly jumping or moving. Others may become overly excited by gross motor play. Vestibular and proprioceptive sensory stimuli affect our level of arousal or activity. Therefore, it is important to observe closely how a child responds to certain forms of vestibular and proprioceptive sensory information. More specific procedures for evaluating vestibular and proprioceptive processing are included in Table 2-11.

Client factors related to neuromusculoskeletal and movement functions.
Evaluation of neuromusculoskeletal components includes assessment of muscle tone, reflexes, postural control and alignment, range of motion, strength, and endurance. Procedures to evaluate muscle tone and postural control are included in Table 2-11, as

Text continues on page 60

TABLE 2-11 | PROCEDURES FOR THE EVALUATION OF PROPRIOCEPTIVE AND VESTIBULAR PROCESSING

Specific Area	Nonstandardized Procedures	Standardized Assessments
Postural control and balance	Evaluation of righting, equilibrium, and protective reactions (Table 3-6); assessment of antigravity movement, including ability to assume and maintain prone extension and supine flexion postures and other developmentally appropriate positions; observations of play activities requiring balance, such as walking on a line or balance beam; playing on suspended equipment such as a platform swing; hopscotch; or riding a bike	MAI (Chandler et al, 1980); AIMS (Piper and Darrah, (1994); BOTMP (Bruininks, 1978); SIPT (Ayres, 1989); TIME (Miller and Roid, 1994); Pediatric Clinical Test of Sensory Interaction for Balance (Horak et al., 1988); (Deitz et al, 1991); DeGangi-Berk Test of Sensory Integration (Berk and DeGangi, 1987)
Muscle tone	Note the amount of resistance felt when muscles are manually lengthened; note the relative softness (low tone) or tension (high tone) in the muscle bellies at rest (usually tested on upper extremities); note any lack of joint mobility (high tone) or hypermobility (low tone), commonly with shoulder flexion/extension, wrist and elbow flexion/extension, hip adduction/abduction, ankle plantar/dorsiflexion	MAI (Chandler et al., 1980); TIME (Miller and Roid, 1994)

| Proprioception | Note whether the child can imitate simple postures and movements; with eyes closed and arms outstretched, test whether the child can bring his or her index finger in to touch his or her nose alternatively with each hand; with eyes closed, move the child's arm in a certain direction and ask the child to replicate the movement with the other arm; note how much the child uses his or her vision to navigate in play and maintain balance | SIPT (Ayres, 1989) |
| Modulation of vestibular and proprioceptive stimuli | Note the child's likes and dislikes for types of movement activity; note the child's response to fast vestibular input (spinning, swinging, jumping) and slow vestibular input (gentle rocking); note the response to heavy pushing and pulling activity (proprioceptive stimuli) | Sensory Profile (Dunn, 1999); The Sensory Rating Scale (Provost and Oetter, 1995); postrotary nystagmus of the SIPT (Ayres, 1989) |

BOTMP, Bruininks-Oseretsky Test of Motor Proficiency; MAI, Movement Assessment of Infants; SIPT, Sensory Integration and Praxis Tests; TIME, Toddler and Infant Motor Evaluation.

they relate to vestibular function, and primitive reflex patterns are discussed in more detail in Chapter 3. Unlike evaluations for adults, formal procedures for evaluating range of motion (ROM) with a goniometer and manual muscle testing to evaluate muscle strength are rarely necessary in an occupational therapy pediatric evaluation. More commonly, these motor components are observed informally, and their impact on functional skill performance is noted.

However, some children may require formal testing of ROM, such as those with limited ROM owing to an orthopedic injury like a hand injury, those with cerebral palsy or traumatic brain injury who are at risk for contractures, and those with juvenile rheumatoid arthritis. Formal testing is important when it is believed that the child's ROM may improve with intervention or when a child may be at risk for losing ROM. Information on conducting formal evaluations of ROM can be found in numerous other sources and therefore is not included herein (see Neistadt, 2000, Trombly, 1995; Gilliam, 1997).

Gross muscle testing evaluates the strength of muscle groups that perform specific movements at each joint, whereas manual muscle testing evaluates the strength of individual muscles. Gross muscle testing might involve observing the child perform sit-ups, push-ups, and knee bends; noting their postural control during gross motor play; or asking the child to move his or her limbs or trunk against resistance. Some standardized assessment tools can also be used, such as Bruininks-Oseretsky Test of Motor Proficiency (Bruininks, 1978), which includes a subtest for measuring muscle strength.

Evaluations of children with certain diagnoses, such as spinal cord injury, neuromuscular dystrophies, and peripheral nerve injuries, may necessitate specific manual muscle testing. To perform muscle testing, you must know the muscles of the body and their functions, the anatomic positions and directions of the muscle fibers, and the angle of pull of the joints. Muscle testing cannot be conducted with children who have abnormal muscle tone. Procedures for conducting manual muscle testing can be found in numerous other sources and therefore are not included herein (see Neistadt, 2000, Trombly, 1995; Simmonds, 1997).

Physical endurance may be evaluated by noting a child's physical tolerance for performing desired or necessary tasks, and it is usually measured by the duration of time a child is able to perform the activity. Endurance is also evaluated by noting the child's postural control over time during activity, reports of fatigue, or need for sleep.

The roles of physical therapists overlap with those of occupational therapists in the evaluation of neuromusculoskeletal functions and motor control. Therefore, at times there may be no need to conduct a thorough evaluation of these factors if these areas have been evaluated by a physical therapist. In addition, physical and occupational therapists may have opportunities to evaluate neuromuscular child factors together. It is, however, important that the functional implications of neuromusculoskeletal problems are clearly documented as part of your occupational therapy evaluation.

Evaluation of Process Skills

Process skills include behaviors that reflect basic mental functions, including cognitive and perceptual skills and social and emotional skills. Generally, process skills are those that we use to plan, initiate, organize, manage, monitor, and modify our actions to complete our daily activities. Communication and interaction skills are addressed as a separate category in the AOTA's Practice Framework (see Appendix A) and therefore are addressed in the next section.

Specific process skills of concern to occupational therapists listed in the AOTA's Practice Framework (see Appendix A) include mental energy or ability to sustain effort; general knowledge and one's ability to select, use, and acquire knowledge; temporal organization and sequencing; organizing space and objects; and the ability to adapt behavior appropriately, such as anticipatory functions and the ability to change behavior in response to feedback. Process skills may be evaluated informally through observations of children completing their daily activities. It is of particular importance for you as the occupational therapist to determine how a child's process abilities and problems are influencing his or her ability to play, make decisions, problem solve, and perform functional or meaningful activities efficiently and safely. The Assessment of Motor and Process Skills (Fisher, 1999) and its School version (Fisher and Bryze, 1997) are examples of standardized assessment tools specifically designed to evaluate process skills.

Client factors that contribute to one's ability to perform process skills include bodily functions and structures related to mental functions, including both global and specific cognitive functions, and psychosocial and emotional skills and behavior. Special education teachers, educational psychologists, and sometimes speech pathologists are professionals with whom you may work who often perform evaluations of cognitive function, including IQ, verbal and nonverbal cognitive skills, speech and language skills, and academic skills testing. As an occupational therapist, you are well trained to evaluate some aspects of mental functioning of children, including psychosocial and emotional development. However, like many other areas of occupational therapy practice, our role in addressing these issues overlap with the roles of other professionals. Clinical child psychologists and psychiatrists focus their evaluations on child mental capacities and behavior, including temperament, personality, and social-emotional development and skills. It is, however, important for you to also evaluate certain mental functions depending on child concerns and the reasons for your evaluation. Normal development of specific cognitive skills and social-emotional development are covered in Chapter 3, and this information provides some guidelines as to the specific cognitive skills and types of behaviors one would expect from children of various ages.

In general, reimbursement for mental health services in the United States often is not as readily available as reimbursement for other service systems (Soloman and Evans, 1992). Therefore, it is important to review records from other professionals addressing psychological issues when they are available and to consult with your team members so that there is a shared understanding of the role of each team member working with a particular child. In preparing for your evaluation of a child with suspected psychological problems, it is important to determine whether any precautions are necessary or whether any specific activities or approaches would be ineffective or counterproductive in your evaluation. When evaluating children and adolescents with a history of behavioral problems, it is important to have some idea of how to approach the child to avoid or minimize difficult or dangerous situations, such as temper outbursts, aggressive behavior, or emotional upset, and to elicit the child's best performance.

In the new AOTA Practice Framework (see Appendix A), mental functions are divided into global and specific types. Global mental functions are more basic functions and include level of consciousness, orientation, sleep, temperament and personality (including emotional stability), and energy/drive (such as motivation and impulse control). Specific mental functions include higher-level cognitive capacities such as judgment, concept formation, calculation ability, sequencing, and use of language. Attention, memory, and perceptual, psychomotor, and emotional functions are also categorized as specific mental functions. Contrary to the AOTA's uniform terminology, which clearly separated psychological and behavioral factors from cognitive functions, under this new system, both cognitive and psychological and behavioral factors are grouped together under the general category of mental functions. Suggested evaluation procedures for global and specific mental functions are described in more detail in the following two subsections.

Evaluation of client factors related to global mental functions. In infants, problems with global mental functions are often associated with a lack of interest in exploring the environment or apathy and with difficulty with sleep and emotional regulation. They may sleep too much, with only short periods of active-alert time, or they may experience difficulty falling asleep, with excessive periods of agitation. Such infants may have difficulty calming down when upset and may cry excessively. Assessment tools aimed at measuring behavioral regulation, including sleep-wake cycles, feeding behavior, sensory preferences, and temperament, are helpful in uncovering global mental impairments in infants and very young children.

Children with traumatic brain injuries or suspected or confirmed mental disorder illness often require more formal evaluations of global mental functions, such as level of consciousness/arousal, orientation, inattention, and emotional regulation and impulse control. The Glascow Coma Scale (see Chapter 4) and Ranchos Levels of Cognitive Functioning (see Neistadt, 2000) are common assessment tools used to evaluate these global mental functions as well as more specific functions such as judgment, memory, and problem-solving ability. Methods of informal evaluation related to cognition for children of various ages are presented in Tables 2-12 and 2-13.

Evaluation of client factors related to specific mental functions. For the purposes of organization, specific mental functions related to psychosocial-emotional functioning are discussed first, followed by specific mental functions relating to cognitive processes. Regardless of the setting in which you work, you will see children with psychosocial and other emotional and behavioral difficulties. Such children may have a documented mental disorder such as attention-deficit hyperactivity disorder or anxiety disorder, or they may be experiencing psychosocial or emotional difficulties in conjunction with other physical or learning disorders. You may be asked to evaluate a child to determine whether he or she fits the diagnostic criteria for a mental disorder, and your occupational therapy evaluation is one piece of information that will contribute to the decision-making/diagnostic process. As discussed in Chapter 1, some occupational therapists work in community health centers and child psychiatric hospitals or residential settings, where the primary concerns of the children they see are related to their mental health, social-emotional development, and behavior.

In addition to record review, common procedures used to evaluate psychosocial skills and other psychological performance components include (1) observations of behavior, particularly naturalistic observations; (2) interviews with the child (often termed a mental status examination) and the caregiver(s); (3) standardized testing, which typically includes questionnaire-type assessment tools that are completed by either the child or a caregiver; and (4) projective activities.

For infants and toddlers, the psychosocial skills and psychological components that you would primarily be

TABLE 2-12	INFORMAL EVALUATION METHODS FOR ASSESSING COGNITIVE SKILLS IN INFANTS AND YOUNG CHILDREN

Cognitive Skill	Informal Evaluation Methods
Ability to recognize familiar vs. new or novel items or persons	Note the child's response (facial expression, reaching behavior) to parents vs. strangers; note the child's interest level with novel vs. familiar toys
Attention/level of arousal/mental energy	Note behavioral cues of alertness, such as facial expressions, and eye focus and tracking during play and interactions; note the length of time the infant or child engages in a particular activity; inquire about the child's typical sleep/awake patterns; note the child's persistence when challenged
Object permanence	Note whether the child will look for a desired hidden object
Adaptation; cause-effect relationships	Note the child's ability to activate cause-effect toys; note anticipatory behavior and ability to learn from errors and to adjust behavior according to environmental cues and feedback
Temporal organization	Note the child's ability to sort shapes and colors and to sort objects with themes, such as animals vs. household objects; note the child's ability to initiate sequence steps and to terminate actions, such as putting toys away where they belong
General knowledge and knowledge of basic concepts	Note the ability of preschool-aged children to sort and identify shapes, colors, and numbers; note their ability to use objects for their intended purpose; note safety judgment and ability to express a desire for assistance
Use of language	Note the child's ability to recognize his or her name, follow simple vs. multi-step directions; note use of expression language (e.g., number of words, length of sentences, ability to express wants)

TABLE 2-13	INFORMAL EVALUATION METHODS FOR ASSESSING COGNITIVE SKILLS IN SCHOOL-AGED CHILDREN AND ADOLESCENTS

Cognitive Skill	**Informal Evaluation Methods**
Orientation x3	Note child's awareness of time, person, and place
Energy and attention	During activity, note the child's ability to attend to and focus on a particular stimulus and the length of time the child is engaged in a specific activity; note the level of persistence when challenged
Memory	Note the child's ability to recall or recognize people or events and to perform tasks that have previously been learned; note the child's ability for new learning by presenting/teaching the child a novel task, such as a computer or card game
Planning, organizing, and sequencing	Note the child's ability to map out a logical, step-by-step approach to multiple tasks and to perform multistep functional activities, such as completing his or her morning self-care routine, getting homework done, keeping his or her desk at school organized and bedroom tidy, and the child's ability to learn and play games with multiple steps and rules
Academics	Ask the child's teacher or parent how the child is performing in academic subjects such as math and reading
Judgment/self-awareness	Note the child's ability to play safely, to identify dangerous situations, and to learn and adhere to safety rules and to be socially appropriate with peers and adults
Problem solving	Note the child's ability to identify problems and viable solutions, to learn novel activities independently, and to learn from errors

concerned with as a part of an occupational therapy evaluation are (1) coping skills, including the ability to demonstrate self-regulatory behaviors; (2) affect and level of interest and engagement in social interactions; (3) the development of healthy attachment behaviors with parents or caregivers; and (4) self-expression and the beginning of development of self-concept. The evaluation of self-regulatory behaviors, temperament, level of interest and engagement in social interactions, self-expression, interests, and self-concept in infants and young children can largely be accomplished through informal observations of the child's play and through caregiver interviews. This evaluation includes observing their interactions with and interest in playing with age-appropriate toys, their social interactions with you, and their interactions with their parents during play. Parents also can provide a wealth of information about their child, including his or her temperament, sleep/wake patterns, attachment behaviors, and ability to cope with stress. Some ways to evaluate attachment behaviors are discussed by Hirshberg (1996). Some standardized assessment tools for measuring infant psychosocial and emotional development are included in Chapter 4 (see Table 4-6).

Naturalistic observations are also very helpful in evaluating psychological components, including social and emotional development, and behavior in preschool and school-aged children. This evaluation may include classroom observations and observation of play and interactions with peers and parents or caregivers. It is important to gain information regarding the child's likes and dislikes; behavior in structured and nonstructured situations; responses to direct requests and challenges; interaction styles with peers, family members, and persons of authority; and coping skills. Parent interviews, as well as interviews with others who care for or see the child on a regular basis (such as teachers), and child interviews are an important part of an evaluation. Interviews with children older than 10 years are particularly helpful for gaining information about the child's values, interests and self-concept, social and interpersonal skills and conduct, coping skills, and self-control. Interviews with children also provide information about their mental status, thought processes, and affect. You may need to refer the child for a more comprehensive and in-depth evaluation by a psychologist or other behavioral specialist when significant concerns are identified.

It is important for you to determine how the child's psychological and cognitive functioning impacts his or her ability to (1) function in important, everyday tasks and activities, such as play and leisure; (2) sustain healthy peer and family relationships; and (3) perform school activities. In addition, it is important to understand the extent to which the child is developing a positive self-image. Specific standardized assessment tools for evaluating psychosocial skills, behavior, and emotional development in preschool- and elementary school-aged children are included in Chapter 4 (see Table 4-6).

As with younger children, the evaluation of psychological, psychosocial, and emotional functioning in adolescents includes observations of behaviors and consideration of important environmental factors such as family and school and relationships with family members, peers, and other important persons in their life.

Observations may be conducted in structured settings, such as during therapeutic group sessions, or in unstructured settings, for example, during a free study period at school. It is important to note how psychosocial, emotional, and other psychological factors are affecting the adolescent's thought processes, feelings about oneself, ability to relate to others, and ability to perform functional activities, school and leisure activities, and any other valued activities.

Incidents like the shootings at Columbine High School in Littleton, Colorado, in 1999 that resulted in the deaths of students and teachers have brought to the forefront the need to determine the potential of individuals to do harm to themselves or others. Interviews with adolescents that include mental status examinations are extremely valuable for extracting information about the student's fears, concerns, coping skills, and feelings about himself or herself and others as well as information about their interests and hopes and dreams for the future.

When individuals have difficulty expressing themselves in words or have suppressed thoughts and feelings, the use of projective techniques or expressive media is often useful (Drake, 1999). Expressive techniques may be used to gain information about self-concept, self-awareness, feelings, and emotions and commonly include a form of drawing or painting but may also include the use of clay, creative writing, or drama or play (Drake, 1999). A list of specific standardized assessment tools to examine this area in adolescents is included in Chapter 4.

Information about the cognitive functions of infants and very young children can be obtained by observing (1) their abilities to recognize familiar versus unfamiliar people and objects and (2) their play with age-appropriate toys that require cognitive skills such as understanding of simple cause-effect, object permanence, spatial concepts, and problem solving. Examples of such toys include "push the button" electronic toys, pop-up toys, different types of puzzles and shape sorter toys, and simple construction toys. Cognitive deficits in preschool children often result in delayed language acquisition and comprehension and in difficulties with play activities that require matching, sorting, and classifying. Preschool children with cognitive deficits may also have motor planning and sequencing difficulties, poor safety judgment, and a general lack of awareness of objects and others in their environment. For example, they may need close supervision or physical assistance to be safe on playground equipment, and they may experience difficulty in learning concepts such as colors, shapes, and numbers and in figuring out ways to play with novel toys or activities.

Some developmental screening tools used by occupational therapists (and other developmental specialists) include cognitive test items such as the Miller Assessment for Preschoolers (Miller, 1988) and the Denver II (Frankenburg and Dodds, 1992). The Bayley Scales of Infant Development (Bayley, 1993) includes a comprehensive scale for measuring mental functions in infants and young toddlers. Attention, judgment, and problem-solving abilities can often be assessed informally by observing children perform age-appropriate functional tasks or play or craft activities. Other methods for informally assessing cognitive functions are included in Tables 2-12 and 2-13.

Evaluation of Communication and Interaction Skills

The AOTA's Practice Framework (see Appendix A) describes communication and interaction skills as the intention, need, and coordination of social behavior to interact with people. These skills include three main areas: physicality or nonverbal communication; information exchange, including the use of language to give and receive information; and the ability to maintain appropriate relationships with others. Speech and language pathologists have expertise in these areas and should be consulted for more thorough evaluations when problems with communication are identified. It is, however, important for you to determine how a child's communication abilities are influencing his or her ability to participate successfully in daily occupations. Normal development of communication abilities and language is described in Chapter 3. This information can be consulted to determine whether infants and young children are achieving major communication, social, and language milestones at the appropriate ages.

Most developmental screening and evaluation tools, such as the Miller Assessment for Preschoolers (Miller, 1988), the Vineland Adaptive Behavior Scales (Sparrow et al., 1984), and the Denver II (Frankenburg and Dodds, 1992), include test items that assess communication or language, and some standardized assessment tools for the evaluation of social skills are included in Chapter 4 (see Table 4-6).

When screening an infant's or toddler's communication and social skills, it is important to note their eye contact, their response to hearing their name and simple directions, and their ability to get their needs and wants known. It is also important to note their spontaneous verbalizations or sounds, their use of words, their use of communicative gestures (such as pointing and waving bye-bye), and their ability to imitate sounds and simple words. In relation to social behavior, observe children for their attachment behaviors and for their comfort level in and preferences for interacting with caregivers and peers versus a preference for being alone.

Once children begin to use language, it is important to note how easily it is to understand what the child is saying (articulation), the length of the utterances (e.g., one- to two-word phrases only), and the functional purposes of the language (to get needs met, to share information and comment, to ask questions, etc.).

For children who use or may benefit from the use of augmentative communication devices, it is important for occupational therapists to analyze the demands (motor and cognitive) of operating a particular device and to determine whether the child has the necessary abilities to operate the device practically and functionally. Complex augmentative communication evaluations conducted to determine the feasibility of using highly technological devices is typically a team process, and the occupational therapy role in this specialized area of evaluation is covered in more detail in Chapter 6.

A child's ability to develop and use language effectively may be affected by underlying cognitive, sensory, motor (particularly oral-motor control and oral praxis), or emotional deficits. Therefore, depending on your hypotheses of why a child may be experiencing problems in this area, you may want to examine further some of the underlying child factors discussed earlier in this chapter. Problems with social skills may also stem from immature social-emotional development or psychological problems, and, if suspected, these child factors should be evaluated in more depth.

STEP 8 Occupational Analysis: Assess Contexts and Activity Demands

Although the **analysis of activity demands** and **contexts** is presented here as a separate step after the analysis of performance skills and client factors, consideration of activity demands and contexts should be made from the time you begin your naturalistic observations and interactions with the child and family, i.e., back in Step 4. It is an ongoing process that can be done throughout Steps 4 through 8.

Context refers to both internal (spiritual and personal belief systems) and external (environmental and sociocultural) contexts and has been described in the Practice Framework as including the following types: cultural, physical, social, personal, spiritual, temporal, and virtual (see Appendix A). Context provides various conditions that sometimes support and sometimes hinder a child's occupational performance. Therefore, when you are trying to identify all of the factors contributing to or affecting a child's ability to participate and succeed in their valued occupations, the context is an essential a part of the evaluation process. It is also an important evaluation component because many contextual elements can be modified to a certain degree. Therefore, an evaluation of contextual factors often leads nicely to intervention planning.

Contextual evaluations are sometimes referred to as ecological evaluations (Neisworth and Bagnata, 1988). Ecological evaluations examine the interaction patterns between individuals and their respective environments, with consideration of physical, social, and cultural influences. It is important not only to gain an understanding of the physical environments and the activities performed within those environments but also to appreciate the basic philosophies of the educational programs attended by the children you are evaluating as well of their religious and cultural backgrounds.

Evaluation of physical, social, and cultural contexts is most often conducted by visual inspection of the environments in which the child is expected to perform his or her daily occupations, such as home, school, child care setting, playground, or work site (for older children). Information about contextual factors can also be obtained through child and caregiver interviews and by reading relevant reference material. Several assessment tools can also be used to elicit this information (see Chapter 4, Table 4-10).

In addition to examining physical environments for accessibility (e.g., maneuverability of wheelchairs and walkers), the child's ability to access toys and materials should be examined. Note the amount and type of visual, auditory, and tactile sensory stimulation or distractions and the organization of materials. Settings for young children should have various toys for both fine motor and gross motor play, imaginative play, and sensory exploration and simple books with large pictures. Such environments should be clean and relatively uncluttered, with child-sized tables and chairs and lowered sinks. Inquire about the child's scheduling of activities (during a school day and during more unstructured time), and examine the environment for its potential to provide opportunities for social interactions and for the child to engage in activities that would promote his or her level of independence or skill development.

An evaluation of activity demands involves examination of the objects, physical space, social demands, sequencing and timing of required actions, and underlying body functions and structures needed to carry out a particular activity (see Appendix A). More simply put, this is the part of your evaluation where you perform a detailed activity analysis on specific tasks or activities that the child you are evaluating is required to do, or wants to do, and that are giving him or her difficulty. Like context, sometimes activity demands can be easily modified to assist a child in being more capable of performing the activity. This would then direct your intervention more to modification of the task or activity than to the child. Generally, activity demands can be identified by observing the child performing the activity in context. As you observe the child, ask (and then answer) the following questions: What are the characteristics of this activity and the steps involved in performing it? What is it about the activity itself that makes it easy or difficult for the child to be successful in performing the activity? Can this activity be done in other ways? How might the activity be modified, or some of the demands eliminated altogether, so that the child could be more successful? More comprehensive processes for conducting activity analyses are provided in most occupational therapy textbooks, such as Willard and Spackman's Occupational Therapy (see Blesedell-Crepeau, 1998).

STEP 9   Conclude Your Evaluation With the Child

Near the end of your evaluation session, you need to determine what you intend to do next, and let the child and family members, nursing staff, or teacher know of your plans. This might include scheduling another appointment to complete the evaluation if you could not gather all the necessary information. You may want to schedule a time to go over the evaluation results with the parent, or if appropriate to your setting, you may plan to have a team meeting with others who work with the child. You may be ready to discuss and develop an intervention plan and then to set up an appointment to begin intervention. More often than not, you will need some time to review all of the evaluation information, to score and interpret any standardized tests, and to pull all of the evaluation data together to begin the intervention planning process. Be sure to thank the child and others who were involved in the evaluation, and commend them on all of their good work. Last, it is important that you document your observations and any other information that you believe is important. Writing down plenty of notes is critical so that you do not forget important information.

STEP 10   Interpret, Synthesize, and Summarize Your
Evaluation Data

After your initial evaluation has been completed and you have scored and interpreted the standardized assessment tools that you administered (see Chapter 4 for guidelines on how to score and interpret standardized tests), you need to synthesize and summarize all of your evaluation data. Some important factors need to be considered when synthesizing evaluation data. Most important, remind yourself of the purpose of the evaluation and of the specific referral questions that were asked of you. By the end of this step you will have clearly addressed the referral questions, with data to support your findings, and will be ready to begin the intervention planning process.

The synthesis of evaluation data from multiple sources specifically for intervention planning is a complex process. The process involves gaining an understanding of the child and family and of the child's ability to participate in his or her valued occupations, as well as a detailed analysis of "why" the child is experiencing difficulty in activities identified as being problematic. Then, this information is used in consideration of service delivery systems, setting, and program considerations to formulate an appropriate intervention plan. More often than not, in pediatrics you will collaborate with other team members during the intervention planning phase so that the most efficient and comprehensive program possible is developed.

The interpretation and synthesis process is broken down further for you into the four-step process outlined in Box 2-2. Each of these four steps is discussed in more detail in the following subsections. Although this process is presented as a series of sequential steps, it is important to note that the last two steps are often carried out simultaneously.

Step One: Formulation of the Occupational Profile

You begin the interpretation, synthesis, and summarization of all of your evaluation data by formulating a brief narrative about the child, an occupational profile. The occupational profile describes who the child is and includes key information such as age; main areas of concern for occu-

---

| **BOX 2-2** | INTERPRETING AND SYNTHESIZING EVALUATION DATA FOR INTERVENTION PLANNING |

Step One: Formulation of the occupational profile. *Who is this child and what are important family characteristics? What are the main presenting problems? What are the primary occupations, including the child's school program and extracurricular activities and interests?*

Step Two: Identification of the child's occupational strengths and challenges. *What areas of occupation (e.g., activities of daily living, education, work, social participation, and play) are presenting challenges for this child? What does this child excel at?*

Step Three: Identification of performance skills and child factors influencing occupational performance. *What specific skills, body functions and structures, and mental capacities are interfering with or supporting the child's ability to perform valued activities? Are you confident that the results of standardized tests reflect the child's true abilities? How does your client's performance compare with that of typical children or children with the same diagnostic condition? How does the child's performance compare with his or her performance in previous evaluations?*

Step Four: Identification of contextual factors and activity demands influencing occupational performance. *How and where is the child expected to perform his or her daily activities, and under what conditions? What objects and actions are required for the child to perform his or her valued activities? What cultural and spiritual factors impact the child's occupational performance? What aspects of the physical environment support or hinder the child's abilities?*

pational therapy; important characteristics of family, school, or child care programs; a summary of the interests and main activities of the child; diagnostic information; and child and family strengths, challenges, and priorities. Samples of occupational profiles are provided in Boxes 2-3, 2-4, and 2-5.

This is not an easy step. The narrative must be concise but include enough information for the reader or listener to develop a basic understanding of the child and why he or she is being seen by an occupational therapist. Most information included in the narrative typically is gained through parent interviews, review of medical and educational records, and informal observations of the child.

Step Two: Identification of the Child's Occupational Strengths and Challenges

Using a top-down approach to evaluation, begin by summarizing the child's ability to perform his or her valued

---

BOX 2-3	SAMPLE OCCUPATIONAL PROFILE: ELEMENTARY SCHOOL–AGED CHILD

Aaron is a 6-year-old boy who was recently diagnosed as having Asperger's syndrome. He lives with his parents and 2-year-old sister. His medical and birth histories are unremarkable, although he does get frequent upper respiratory tract infections. Developmental milestones were reported to be achieved within the age-appropriate ranges, including walking at 13 months of age and saying his first words at 16 months. Toilet training was challenging and was completed when he was 3 and a half years of age. Aaron attends a regular half-day kindergarten program, and he is currently being evaluated to determine whether he requires special education services. He was referred for an occupational therapy evaluation because of difficulties with fine motor skills and suspected sensory processing problems. His parents and teacher are particularly concerned about his inability to adapt to change, the frequency and intensity of temper outbursts, and his emotional reactivity in general; they feel that his play behaviors and social skills are very immature. Aaron likes to play with dinosaur action figures and computers, and he is an avid fan of Nickelodeon TV shows. He is currently taking swimming lessons, and he has many children to play with in his neighborhood, although he usually chooses to play on his own. Both parents work outside the home, and Aaron's grandmother baby-sits him and his sister while they are at work.

BOX 2-4	SAMPLE OCCUPATIONAL PROFILE: ADOLESCENT

Ray is an 18-year-old senior in high school. He lives with his 12-year-old brother and his parents in a rural community. Ray is an excellent student and an active member of the National Honor Society; he has been accepted to attend university in the Fall on a full scholarship in computer technologies. Ray has type II spinal muscular atrophy. His disease process has been slowly progressive. He has little active movement or strength in his lower extremities, and he currently uses a perm-mobile, power wheelchair that reclines, raises, and lowers as his means of mobility. He has a custom lap tray to support his driving, computer, and other classroom needs. Ray requires maximal assistance for all transfers and for dressing, bathing, and toileting. He can do most simple grooming activities and can eat independently with setup. Ray needs help with positioning at night, and he requires oxygen at night. At school, he keeps up by using his laptop computer for taking notes. He mainly uses the keyboard for software navigation because using the mouse is too fatiguing for him. Outside of school, Ray has a part-time job as a Web page designer, and he volunteers at a retirement community where he helps residents learn how to use computers. He is an avid soccer fan. Ray has a very supportive family, but he is excited about leaving home and going off to college in the near future.

occupations (e.g., instrumental ADLs, play, school activities). What are the important functional skills that the child is experiencing difficulty with? What can the child do well? The AOTA's Practice Framework (2002, XVIII, final draft) (see Appendix A), includes the following areas of occupation that may be important to address in your evaluation: ADLs, such as bathing and eating; instrumental ADLs, such as care of pets, communication device use, and shopping; education or school participation; work; play; leisure; and social participation with family, peers, and friends and with community members and agencies.

Results from functional assessments such as the Pediatric Evaluation of Disability Inventory (Haley et al.,1992) and the School Function Assessment (Coster et al., 1998) are helpful in summarizing a child's ability to perform functional activities. Consider the priorities discussed by the child, the child's parents, and other significant individuals (e.g., the child's teacher). What are the most important roles and activities the child is involved in that are posing problems? This information helps you, as the occupational

BOX 2-5	SAMPLE OCCUPATIONAL PROFILE: INFANT

Molly is a 3-month-old infant (chronologic age) with a corrected age of 1 month. She was born prematurely at 32 weeks' gestation, largely as a result of maternal drug abuse. Molly lives with her mother and maternal grandmother, who both receive social assistance. She has two sisters, 5 and 6 years of age, who also reside in the home. All the children have different fathers, and only the eldest has regular contact with her father. Molly's mother is being treated as an outpatient for substance abuse, and she has a history of bipolar disorder. Her grandmother assumes the role of primary caregiver for all of the children, although their mother is also very involved and seems motivated to enhance her parenting skills and take on more of the responsibility. They live in a small home with plenty of toys.

Molly was hospitalized for 6 weeks after she was born. Results of infant and mother urinalysis for perinatal cocaine were positive. Her birth weight was 1,600 g, and her Apgar scores were 5 and 7 at 1 and 5 minutes, respectively. While hospitalized, she developed respiratory distress syndrome and experienced feeding difficulties and failure to thrive. She also had state regulation problems characterized by diffuse sleep and frequent agitation when awake. These problems gradually decreased. At hospital discharge, Molly was drinking adequately from the bottle, although she continued to be irritable and difficult to calm. She is currently being evaluated by the county early intervention services.

therapist, determine the important functional areas to address in an intervention program. These areas are often used to develop the child's functional long-term intervention goals. For example, in a hospital setting, you might generate a problem list that includes the areas of mobility, social and play skills, and feeding for a child who demonstrated difficulties performing these occupations and when improvements in these areas were found to be important to the child and parents.

Step Three: Identification of Performance Skills and Child Factors Influencing Occupational Performance

The results of tests designed to measure specific child factors and performance skills provide information about why a child may or may not be able to engage successfully in their daily occupations. As discussed earlier in this chapter, the analysis of occupational performance involves evaluation of motor, process, and communication skills. Client or child (for our purposes) factors relate directly to the physiologic and structural functions of the body. For example, an examination of mental functions may help us answer such questions as the following: Are underlying memory or organizational difficulties contributing to the child's difficulty with making transitions between classes at school? Specific evaluations of motor functions may help us determine whether the child has neuromuscular problems, such as decreased joint mobility, abnormal muscle tone, or muscle weakness, that affect his or her gross motor play. Recall that your decision to administer assessment tools measuring performance skills and specific client factors was based on your hypothesis that some of these child factors and performance skills were probably contributing to the child's difficulty in performing functional activities. Therefore, results of standardized tests often help identify some of the underlying factors or "why" a child is experiencing difficulty with a particular type of task. Scores from norm-referenced tests also provide a comparison of your client's underlying skills with that of typical children of the same or a similar age and can elicit information about the degree or severity of a child's problem.

When interpreting the results of standardized tests, it is important to consider how valid you believe the child's scores are. Did you administer the test in the standardized way in which it was intended to be administered? Was the child able to understand the directions? How valid and reliable is the assessment tool itself? Did the child put forth his or her best effort? It is important to include a statement about your confidence with respect to the extent to which test scores reflect the child's true abilities. Were the test results consistent with parent reports of performance and with your informal observations?

Next, consider evaluation information gained from formal and informal observations. Apply your knowledge of normal child development and what you expect of children at various ages. Begin to identify how the children's strengths, challenges, or deficit areas seem to influence their abilities to perform valued activities or occupations, such as self-care skills, school-related activities, or play activities. This is particularly important in school settings, where legislation (the Individuals With Disabilities Education Act [1997]) requires that related service providers such as occupational therapists demonstrate how children's areas of difficulty and intervention goals relate directly to their ability to perform school activities.

This step ends by identifying and describing the extent of specific performance skills and child factors that are contributing to the child's difficulties in performing his or her daily occupations. Many of these skills and child factors may be the areas that are addressed as part of the occupational therapy intervention program that you will develop. Some of these areas will be addressed by other team members. Others may not be addressed at all if it is believed that they cannot be significantly altered or when there are other priorities or means by which the child can learn to successfully engage in the challenging occupations. In most settings, you would include some of these skills and factors as a part of the child's problem list, or list of challenges, which, as noted previously, reflects some of the areas that you ultimately would like to address in an occupational therapy program. Finally, it is important to note the child factors and skills that represent the child's strengths because strengths need to be considered, and capitalized on, as you develop your intervention plan.

Step Four: Identification of Contextual Factors and Activity Demands Influencing Occupational Performance

Concurrently with the interpretation of information related to child factors, you will identify the contextual factors, including sociocultural, spiritual, and environmental contexts, and activity demands that are most salient in supporting or hindering the child's ability to engage successfully in his or her daily occupations. As you attempt to uncover the reasons why a child is or is not experiencing success, consider the opportunities the child has had to develop certain skills. What are the sociocultural expectations, values, and priorities that have been influential in the child's development and that continue to be an integral part of their lives? For occupational therapists to assist children in interacting successfully with individuals and objects in their environments and meeting the everyday demands placed on them, it is important that such contextual factors are identified and reported. For example, when evaluating a school-aged child with academic problems, learning about his or her curriculum; the physical classroom environment; the teacher's style, philosophy, and expectations of children in the classroom; and parental attitudes toward school achievement are all necessary for you to make effective recommendations for improving the child's ability to perform classroom activities. The analysis of contexts and activity demands involves the synthesis of information primarily from ecological assessment tools; observations of physical environments, including space, equipment, and materials; observations of the child performing activities in natural contexts; and caregiver and child interviews.

Contextual factors are particularly important to consider during the evaluation of ADLs, such as feeding, which are often heavily influenced by sociocultural factors. Parenting practices are also culturally sensitive and have a direct impact on child behavior. Once contextual factors are examined, they need to be considered in your interpretations of standardized test results and when interpreting your formal and informal observations. Finally, contextual information is vital to consider as you formulate your intervention plans to ensure that programming suggestions make sense to the children and families that are referred, are practical and address the areas that are most valued, and, finally, are delivered in ways that best fit or match their contextual lives.

STEP 11 Develop Recommendations and Intervention Planning

The initial evaluation process ends with the development and documentation of recommendations and, when appropriate, the development of an occupational therapy intervention plan. Typically, an intervention plan is not necessary when the purpose of the evaluation was consultative in nature (conducted to provide recommendations around a specific problem area) or when the evaluation yielded results indicating that the child does not require occupational intervention services. In both cases, however, recommendations should still be provided, including helpful suggestions for enhancing the child's ability to successfully engage in his or her daily occupations. In addition, referrals for other services or evaluations may be suggested when appropriate.

Developing an intervention plan involves the synthesis of all your evaluation data, with setting, system, and program factors and other practical considerations. As noted earlier, it is rare that you would create an occupational therapy intervention program in isolation. Instead, you would collaborate with the child, parents or caregivers, teachers, and other members of the child's team. Sometimes your program planning efforts will be used to create one interdisciplinary or transdisciplinary educational, rehabilitation, or family services program. Other times, depending on your setting, you may create your own individual occupational therapy program. However, even when creating a separate occupational therapy intervention plan, it is best practice to gain a general understanding of the other services a child is receiving to avoid unnecessary duplication of services and to facilitate consistent approaches when it would be helpful to do so.

The intervention planning process includes the development of long-term goals and short-term, measurable objectives. You have the complex task of selecting from various specific frames of reference and intervention techniques available to occupational therapists. You also may have several service delivery options (indirect versus direct services and working with a certified occupational therapist assistant or rehabilitation aide) available to you from which to choose. Some factors that you will need to consider as you begin to make intervention planning decisions are the level of research evidence supporting the interventions that you are considering, client preferences, available equipment and materials, and your own skill level. In addition to writing intervention goals and objectives, your intervention plan must include a schedule, with the lengths and times of sessions noted, and the projected functional outcomes of your interventions need to be identified. This book does not go into detail with respect to occupational therapy intervention services. However, the intervention planning process is covered in detail in Chapter 7, including information and specific examples on how to write goals and objectives.

STEP 12   Document and Share Your Evaluation Results

The final step in the evaluation process includes documentation of the evaluation and sharing of the information. After every evaluation session you have with a client, it is important for you to document at a minimum the time you spent with the client, a summary of the evaluation activities that you completed, and your next plan of action. In a medical setting, this kind of note is typically entered in the progress note section of the medical chart. In school- or community-based settings, you may have your own client files that you keep, and a note would be entered in that file.

Various sample outlines for writing pediatric occupational therapy evaluations for different practice settings and types of children are provided in Chapter 7. As you will see, individual styles and preferences can be applied to the writing of reports. However, it is important that you check with your supervisor to determine the acceptable formats for evaluation reports in your setting. At minimum, the following information should be included in any occupational therapy evaluation of children:

- Demographic data (child's name, date of birth, age, parents' names, address, and telephone number)
- School information, when applicable (grade, school program, and teacher)
- Referring information (referral source, reasons for referral, child's primary physician)
- A description of the evaluation methods and tests used
- An occupational profile (background information, including relevant medical history; the child's occupations, interests, and valued activities; a description of family and other important relationships; and a brief description of school and extracurricular or work activities)

- A description of the child's behavior during the evaluation (e.g., mood, affect, ability to follow directions, attention, activity level, activity preferences, and effort)
- Evaluation results, including test scores and a summary of clinical and naturalistic observations and interview data (including information on the child's ability to perform his or her daily occupations and on the performance skills, client factors, and contextual and activity factors that support or hinder participation in valued occupations)
- An evaluation summary and impressions (e.g., child strengths and challenges, child and family priorities, contextual factors, and the need for further services from an occupational therapist or others)
- Recommendations (intervention plans, referrals, etc.)
- Your name, signature, and qualifications and the date of the evaluation

In addition to communicating your evaluation results in written format, you will need to share your results with other professionals who work with the child, the referral source, and the parents and, when applicable, the child. It is important that you use appropriate language for your audience so that your evaluation results are easily understood and can be verbally presented in a concise and clear manner.

FINAL THOUGHTS AND HELPFUL HINTS TO CONSIDER THROUGHOUT THE EVALUATION PROCESS

When following a client-centered practice model, it is always necessary to put the clients' needs ahead of your own. There will be times when you cannot complete your planned evaluation activities owing to unforeseen scheduling conflicts, family or child illness, or child behavioral concerns. Sometimes you may administer only part of a standardized test before needing to stop because the child being evaluated is uncomfortable or is experiencing difficulty following the directions. Do not panic. You have gained a lot of information about the child by attempting to administer the test, and getting test scores is not the most important part of your evaluation. Remember that your role is to help your clients, and sometimes that may mean foregoing most of your well-thought-out evaluation plan and being flexible enough to adapt, sometimes "on the spot," to the needs of the child and family. It is not always possible to anticipate exactly what you will need to do and what materials and equipment you will need. Thinking about a "backup plan" ahead of time is a helpful practice.

Second, be aware of the reliability and validity and the strengths and limitations of the assessment tools and procedures you are using. You want to select the most helpful evaluation methods and assessments tools and complete your evaluation efficiently and in the way that is least taxing on all of the individuals that you will involve in the evaluation process. Efficiency is significantly enhanced when preevaluation activities (such as record reviews and interviews) are thorough and when information gathered from other professionals is shared (avoiding duplication).

Third, be careful not to confuse your direct observations of behavior with your interpretations of behavior as you synthesize evaluation data and document your evaluation. This is a common mistake made by professionals. Be clear to distinguish in your documentation what you "saw" or how the child "scored" on a test from your interpretations of the score or the behavior. This process is covered in more depth in Chapter 5.

Finally, be timely in getting your evaluation results interpreted and your report delivered to the necessary individuals. The results of your evaluation are important to the child and family and often will have direct implications on the kinds of programming and interventions that a child will receive or is receiving.

SUMMARY

The purpose of this chapter was to take you through a 12-step occupational therapy evaluation process for children by directly applying the Practice Framework adopted by the AOTA in May 2002. This evaluation process follows a top-down approach and includes the development of an occupational profile of the child you are evaluating, followed by a detailed analysis of the child's occupational performance. The analysis of occupational performance includes evaluation of child factors, including motor, process, and communication skills, and evaluation of contextual and activity demand elements. The importance of relating child factors and contextual and activity demand factors to the child's success in performing his or her valued occupations is emphasized and will be one of the ways in which your occupational therapy evaluation will be distinguished from the evaluations from other disciplines.

Chapters 3 provides an overview of normal development and is included as supplemental resource information to assist you in selecting appropriate evaluation materials, toys, and activities for children of various ages and to guide you in interpreting your informal observations. The remaining chapters provide detailed information and practical examples to assist you in completing the more complex steps of this evaluation process.

References

American Occupational Therapy Association (2002). Occupational Therapy Practice Framework: Domain and process. *American Journal of Occupational Therapy, 56,* 609–639.

American Occupational Therapy Association (1994). Uniform terminology for occupational therapy—third edition. *American Journal of Occupational Therapy, 49,* 1029–1031.

American Psychiatric Association (1994). Diagnostic and statistical manual of mental disorders (4th ed.). Washington, DC: Author.

Amundson, S.J. (1995). *Evaluation tool of children's handwriting (ETCH).* Homer, AK: O.T. Kids Inc..

Ayres, A.J. (1989). *Sensory integration and praxis tests.* Los Angeles, CA: Western Psychological Services.

Baron & Curtin (1999). Reliability of the self–assessment of occupational functioning, *American Journal of Occupational Therapy, 53(5),* 482–488.

Bayley, N. (1993). *Bayley scales of infant development* (2nd ed.). San Antonio, TX: The Psychological Corp.

Beery, K. (1997). *Beery-Buktenica developmental test of visual-motor integration (VMI),* (4th ed.). Parsippany, NJ: Modern Curriculum Press.

Berk, R., DeGangi, G. (1987). *DeGangi-Berk test of sensory integration*. Los Angeles, CA: Western Psychological Services.

Black, M. (1976). Adolescent role assessment. *American Journal of Occupational Therapy 30*, 73–79.

Blesedell-Crepeau, E. (1998). Activity analysis: A way of thinking about occupational performance. In M.E. Neistadt & E.B. Crepeau (Eds.), *Willard & Spackman's occupational therapy* (9th ed., pp. 135–148). Philadelphia, PA: Lippincott Williams & Wilkins.

Brasic-Royeen, C.B., & Fortune, J.C. (1990). TIE: Touch inventory for school-aged children. *American Journal of Occupational Therapy, 44*, 155–160.

Brasic-Royeen, C.B., & Lane, S. (1991). Tactile processing and sensory defensiveness. In A. Fisher, E. Murray, & A. Bundy (Eds.), *Sensory integration theory and practice* (pp. 108–133). Philadelphia, PA: F.A. Davis Co.

Brown, C., & Dunn, W. (2002). *Sensory profile: Adolescent/adult version*. San Antonio, TX: The Psychological Corporation.

Bruininks, R.H. (1978). *Bruininks-Oseretsky test of motor proficiency*. Circle Pines, MN: American Guidance Service.

Caldwell, B.M., & Bradley, R.H. (1984). *Home observation for the measurement of the environment–revised*. Little Rock, AK: University of Arkansas.

Chandler, L., Andrews, M., & Swanson, M. (1980). *Movement assessment of infants*. Rolling Bay, WA: Chandler, Andrews, and Swanson.

Colarussi, R., & Hammill, D. (1995). *The motor free visual perception test–revised*. Novato, CA: Academic Therapy Publications.

Cooper, J., Majnerner, A., Rosenblatt, B., & Birnbaum, R. (1993). A standardized sensory assessment for children of school-age. *Physical and Occupational Therapy in Pediatrics, 13*(1), 61–80.

Coulton, C.J. (1979). Developing an instrument to measure person-environment fit. *Journal of Social Service Research, 3*, 159–173.

Coster, W., Deeney, T., Haltiwanger, J., & Haley, S. (1998). *School Function Assessment (SFA)*. San Antonio, TX: Psychological Corp.

DeGangi, G. A., & Greenspan, S.I (1989). *Test of sensory function in infants*. Los Angeles, CA: Western Psychological Services.

Deitz, J., Richardson, P., Atwater, S., & Odiome, M. (1991). Performance of children on the pediatric clinical test of sensory integration for balance. *The Occupational Therapy Journal of Research, 7*(6), 336–356.

Dematteo, C., Law, M., Russell, D., Pollack, N., Rosenbaum, P., & Walter, S. (1993). The reliability and validity of the quality of upper extremity skills test. *Physical and Occupational Therapy in Pediatrics, 13*(2), 1–18.

Drake, M. (1999). The use of expressive media as an assessment tool in mental health. In B. Hemphill-Pearson's (Ed.), *Assessments in mental health: An integrative approach* (pp. 129–137). Thorofare NJ: Slack, Inc.

Dubowitz, L., & Dubowitz, V. (1981). *The neurological assessment of the preterm and full term newborn infant. Clinics in Developmental Medicine, No. 79.* Philadelphia, PA: J.B. Lippincott.

Dunn, W. (1999). *Sensory profile, user's manual.* San Antonio, TX: The Psychological Corporation.

Erhardt, R.P. (1989). *Erhardt developmental vision assessment.* Tucson, AZ: Therapy Skill Builders.

Erhardt, R.P. (1994). *Developmental prehension assessment–revised.* San Antonio, TX: Psychological Corp.

Fisher, A.G. (1999). *Assessment of motor and process skills* (3rd ed). Fort Collins, CO: Three Star Press.

Fisher, A.G., & Bryze K. (1997). *School AMPS: School version of the assessment of motor and process skills.* Fort Collins, CO: Three Star Press.

Fisher, A.G. (1994). *Assessment of motor and process skills manual* (research edition 7.0) Unpublished test manual. Fort Collins, CO: Colorado State University.

Fisher, A.G. (1991). Vestibular-proprioceptive processing and bilateral integration and sequencing deficits. In A. Fisher, E. Murray, & A. Bundy (Eds.), *Sensory integration theory and practice* (pp. 71–104). Philadelphia, PA: F.A. Davis Co.

Folio, R., & Fewell, R. (2000). *Peabody developmental motor scales–2* (2nd ed.). Austin, TX: Pro-Ed.

Frankenburg, W.K., & Dodds, J. (1992). *Denver II, screening manual.* Denver, CO: Denver Developmental Materials, Inc.

Furuno, S., O'Reilly, K., Hosaka, C.M., Zeisloft, B., & Allman, T. (1984). *The Hawaii early learning profile.* Palo Alto, CA: VORT.

Gardner, M. (1995). *Test of visual-motor skills–revised.* Hydesville, CA: Psychological and Educational Publications Inc.

Gardner, M. (1997). *Test of visual-perceptual skills (non-motor)–revised.* Hydesville, CA: Psychological and Educational Publications Inc.

Gilliam, J. (1997). Joint range of motion. In J. Van Deusen, & D. Brunts (Eds.), *Assessment in occupational therapy and physical therapy* (pp. 49–77). Philadelphia, PA: W.B. Saunders Company.

Griswold, L. (1994). Ethnographic analysis: A study of classroom environments. *American Journal of Occupational Therapy, 48*(5), 397–402.

Hagen, C. (1998). *Ranchos levels of cognitive function. A clinical case management tool* (3rd ed.). Escondido, CA: Author.

Hamilton, B.B., & Granger, C.U. (1991). *Functional independence measure for children (Wee-FIM)*. Buffalo, NY: Research Foundation of the State University of New York.

Haley, S., Coster, W., Ludlow, L., Haltiwanger, J., & Andrellos, P. (1992). *Pediatric evaluation of disability inventory*. San Antonio, TX: Psychological Corp.

Hirshberg, L. (1996). History-making, not history-taking: Clinical interviews with infants and their families. In S. Mesisel & E. Fenichel's (Eds.), *New visions for the developmental assessment of infants and young children* (pp. 85–124). National Center for Infants and Toddlers: Zero to Three.

Horak, F.B., Shumway-Cook, A., Crowe, T.K., Black F.O. (1988). Vestibular function and motor proficiency in children with impaired hearing, or with learning disability and motor impairments. *Developmental Medicine and Child Neurology, 30,* 64–79.

Individuals with Disabilities Education Act (IDEA) Amendments of 1997 (PL.105-17). U.S.C. 1400.

Klein, R., & Bell, B. (1982). *Klein-Bell ADL scale*. Seattle, WA: University of Washington, HSCER Distribution.

Knox, S. (1997). Development and current use of the Knox Preschool Play Scale. In L.D. Parham & L.S. Fazio (Eds.), *Play in occupational therapy* (pp. 35–51). St Louis, MO: Mosby.

Law, M., Baptiste, S., Carswell, A., McColl, M., Polatajko, H., & Pollock, N. (1994). Canadian Occupational Performance Measure. Toronto, Ontario, CAN: The Canadian Association of Occupational Therapists.

Logemann, J.A. (1983). *Evaluation and treatment of swallowing disorders*. San Diego, CA: College Hill Press.

Matthews, P.B. (1988). Proprioceptors and their contribution to somatosensory mapping: Complex messages require complex mapping. *Canadian Journal of Physiology and Pharmacology, 66,* 430–438.

Miller, L.J. (1988). *Miller assessment for preschoolers*. San Antonio, TX: Psychological Corporation.

Miller, L.J., & Roid, G.H. (1994). *The T.I.M.E. Toddler and Infant Motor Evaluation: A standardized assessment*. Tucson, AZ: Therapy Skill Builders.

Morris, S.E., & Klein, M.D. (1987). *Pre-feeding skills*. Tucson, AZ: Therapy Skill Builders.

Neisworth, J.T., & Bagnata, S.J. (1988). Assessment in early childhood education: A typology of dependent measures. In S.L. Odom & M.B. Karnes (Eds.), *Early intervention for infants and children with handicaps: An empirical base* (pp. 23–49). Baltimore, MD: P.H. Brookes.

Neistdadt, M. (2000). *Occupational therapy evaluation for adults: A pocket guide*. Philadelphia, PA: Lippincott Williams & Wilkins.

Piers, E.V. (1984). *Piers-Harris children's self-concept scale (revised manual)*. Los Angeles, CA: Western Psychological Services.

Piper, M. & Darrah, J. (1994). *Motor assessment of the developing infant*. Philadelphia, PA: W.B. Saunders.

Provost, B., & Oetter, P. (1995). The sensory rating scale for infants and young children: Development and reliability. *Physical and Occupational Therapy in Pediatrics, 13*(4), 15–35.

Richter, E., & Montgomery, P. (1991). *The sensorimotor performance analysis*. Hugo, MN: PDP Products.

Rogers, J.C., & Holm, M.B. (1998). Evaluation of activities of daily living (ADL) and home management. In M.E. Neistadt & E.B. Crepeau (Eds.), *Willard & Spackman's occupational therapy* (9th ed., pp. 185–208). Philadelphia, PA: Lippincott Williams & Wilkins.

Russell, D., Rosenbaum, P., Gowland, C., Hardy, S., Lane, M., Plews, N., Mc Gavin, H., Cadman, D., & Jarvis, S. (1993). *Gross motor function measure–revised*. Owen Sound, Ontario, Canada: Pediatric Physiotherapy Services.

Scheiman, M. (1991). *Pediatric clinical vision screening for occupational therapists*. Philadelphia, PA: Pennsylvania College of Optometry.

Simmonds, M. (1997). Muscle strength. In J. Van Deusen & D. Brunts (Eds.), *Assessment in occupational therapy and physical therapy* (pp. 27–48). Philadelphia, PA: W.B. Saunders Company.

Solomon, P., & Evans, D. (1992). Service needs of youths released from a state psychiatric facility as perceived by service provider and families. *Community Mental Health Journal, 28*, 305–315.

Sparrow, S., Balla, D., & Cicchetti, D. (1984). *The Vineland adaptive behavior scales, interview edition: Survey form manual*. Circle Pines, MN: American Guidance Service.

Trombly, C.A. (1995). Evaluation of biomechanical and physiological aspects of motor performance. In C. A. Trombly (Ed.), *Occupational therapy for physical dysfunction* (4th ed., pp.73–156). Baltimore: Williams & Wilkins.

Trombly, C.A., & Quintana, L.A. (1989). Activities of daily living. In C.A. Trombly (Ed.), *Occupational therapy for physical dysfunction* (3rd ed., pp. 386–410). Baltimore: Williams & Wilkins.

World Health Organization (1998). International Classification of Impairments, disabilities and handicaps: A manual of classification relating to the consequences of disease. Geneva: World Health Organization.

Zerilli, K.S., Stefans, V.A., & DiPietro, M.A. (1990). Protocol for the use of videofluoroscopy in pediatric swallowing dysfunction. *The American Journal of Occupational Therapy, 44* (5), 441–446.

3
TYPICAL CHILD DEVELOPMENT

INTRODUCTION

The purpose of this chapter is to provide you with some basic information regarding normal or typical child development. Knowledge of current concepts and theories related to child development is essential for you as an occupational therapist to be competent in conducting evaluations of children. This background information provides a rationale for explaining why you are evaluating what you are evaluating, helps with your interpretation of information gathered, and also provides some guidance as you get ready to develop your intervention plans for children.

The chapter begins by introducing you to some basic theory related to normal development and to occupational therapy. Second, the most common occupations of children are examined with an emphasis on when and how children of various ages typically experience or engage in these everyday occupations. The occupations discussed include play and leisure skills, instrumental and basic activities of daily living, school activities, and family, peer, and community relationships and participation. Third, the typical underlying skills and capacities acquired by infants and children at various ages in several developmental areas are presented because these skills influence the ways in which children engage in developmentally appropriate tasks and activities. The developmental areas discussed include motor development (fine, gross, and oral-motor skills), cognitive skills, language and communication skills, and psycho-emotional and social development.

DEVELOPMENTAL PRINCIPLES AND THEORIES

Background knowledge in theories of occupational therapy and of child development will help you make decisions as you formulate your evaluation and intervention plans for children. **Developmental theories** have been, and continue to be, developed to clearly describe and organize child behavior and to provide insights from which one can make predictions of behavior. Theories of development attempt to explain the qualitative changes, both physical and psychological, experienced by children as they move from infancy through childhood to adulthood. Some theories are global, whereas others focus on explaining changes that occur over time in specific areas of development, e.g., cognition and social-emotional development. In addition, theories are used to help explain important concepts related to development, e.g., the roles of **nature versus nurture, resiliency and vulnerability, individual differences,** and the **relationships among various domains of development**. Different theories are not discussed in this chapter in any detail; therefore, you will need to refer to other resources for more in-depth discussion of and information on this topic. However, some basic principles regarding development that are universally accepted are presented in Box 3-1. Table 3-1 describes some of the most prominent developmental theories that you should be familiar with.

For your occupational therapy evaluations to be consistent with the philosophy, values, and domains of concern of our profession, they should be based on an **occupation-based theoretical model**. Several frameworks focus on occupational performance by emphasizing one's ability to engage successfully in his or her valued daily activities or occupations. Occupation-based theoretical models, such as the Model of Human Occupation (Kielhofner, 1995), the Person-Environment-Performance

| **BOX 3-1** | GENERAL DEVELOPMENTAL PRINCIPLES |

1. Development depends on the interaction of three main factors: (a) genetic predisposition; (b) the individual's own role in his or her development, including previous experience or developmental history; and (c) environmental factors (family and sociocultural). The relative importance of each of these factors and how they interact with one another to influence development are controversial among theorists.

2. The areas of development (e.g., motor and language) are interdependent. However, the nature of the interaction among areas of development is poorly understood.

3. Most aspects of development progress toward greater complexity or advancement via a gradual, continuous process. Some aspects of development are believed to progress through specific stages in which there are periods of rapid growth during transitions between stages, followed by more stable periods, when little change occurs.

4. Sensitive or critical periods exist for some areas of development. These are brief periods during which the neonate or developing child is particularly vulnerable or highly responsive to specific kinds of environmental experiences or stimuli.

5. Development progresses toward a state of homeostasis or balance via a process of adaptation to challenge or stress.

Adapted from Angoff W. The nature-nurture debate, aptitude and group differences. Am Psychol 1988;43:713–720; Bayley N. Bayley Scales of Infant Development (BSID-II). San Antonio, TX: The Psychological Corporation, 1993; Bukatko D, Daehler M. Child Development: A Thematic Approach. Boston: Houghton Mifflin Co, 2001; Case-Smith J. Development of childhood occupations. In: Case-Smith J, ed. Occupational Therapy for Children. 4th Ed. St Louis: Mosby, 2001:71–94; Gormly A, Brodzinsky D. Lifespan Human Development. 5th Ed. Fort Worth: Harcourt Brace Jovanovich Publishers, 1993; and Sroufe LA, Cooper RG, DeHart GB. Child Development: Its Nature and Course. 2nd Ed. New York: McGraw-Hill, 1992.

Model (Christiansen and Baum, 1997), the Ecology of Human Performance (Dunn et al., 1994), and the Person-Environment-Occupation Model (Law et al., 1996), emphasize the importance of considering client factors (the skills and abilities of the individual) as well as the contextual factors and task demands within which the occupations are performed (Case-Smith, 2001; also see the American Occupational Therapy Association's (AOTA's) Occupational Therapy Practice Framework (AOTA, 2002).

TABLE 3-1 THEORETICAL PERSPECTIVES ON DEVELOPMENT

Theory	Description	References
Learning theory approaches	Outgrowth of behaviorism; emphasizes social and emotional development; learning is believed to occur through observation and then imitation of behavior (modeling) and through experience with positive and negative consequences; includes behaviorist approaches, e.g., applied behavioral analysis and social learning theory	Skinner, 1957; Bandura, 1977; Gewirtz and Pelaez-Nogueras, 1992
Psychoanalytic and psychosocial theories	These theories focus on personality, social, and emotional development; Freudian theory includes five psychosexual stages and supports the notion that behavior is largely influenced by inner primitive drives and instincts; Erikson's theory modified Freudian principles by emphasizing the psychological issues that need to be addressed at each of eight stages of psychosocial development	Freud, 1966; Erikson, 1963; Bukatko and Daehler, 2001
Theories of cognitive development	Emphasizes how children of different ages think, adapt to, organize, and interpret their experiences; generally assumes that healthy children have similar mental, social, and emotional capacities; also includes motor learning theory	Flavell, 1996; Piaget, 1971; Case, 1995; Schmidt, 1988

Information processing	Emphasizes the development of cognitive skills, particularly those related to attention, memory, thinking skills, and problem solving abilities; views humans as having a limited capacity to process information	Seigler, 1983a, b; Krantz, 1994; Massaro and Cowan, 1993
Maslow's Hierarchy of Needs	Developed a hierarchy of human needs, proposing that the most basic needs (such as food and shelter) must be met before intellectual or emotional, self-fulfilling needs	Cited by Hall and Lindzey, 1978
Contextual approaches	System views emphasizing the influences of one's sociocultural physical, historical, and spiritual contexts on development; includes ecologic systems perspectives, dynamic systems theory, and Vygotsky's sociohistorical theory	Bukatko and Daehler, 2001; Vygotsky, 1978; Bronfenbrenner and Ceci, 1994
Adaptational theory	Addresses social, emotional, and cognitive aspects of development	Bowlby, 1982

The application of a top-down model for evaluation encourages you to first evaluate the performance of children in their valued roles and occupations. The occupations of a particular child largely define who he or she is. Typically, **occupations of children** include play and leisure; instrumental and basic activities of daily living; school activities; family, peer, and community relationships and participation; and prevocational and vocational activities. **Occupational performance** refers to one's ability to successfully engage in his or her chosen occupations, and this ability depends on three interconnected factors: individual abilities; the occupations themselves, including the demands of the specific tasks and activities associated with the occupations; and contexts (Case-Smith, 2001).

Throughout the occupational therapy evaluation process, theoretical information assists you in selecting appropriate assessment tools and activities, formulating important and relevant interview questions for teachers and caregivers, and guiding your informal observations (i.e., what you should be looking for in children of certain ages). A strong foundation of knowledge of normal development will also assist you in interpreting your evaluation data and in providing appropriate interventions.

OCCUPATIONS OF CHILDHOOD

Play and Leisure

It is primarily through play that infants and young children learn and practice new skills and refine others, experiment with social roles, experience emotions, and develop friendships. Children are intrinsically motivated to play, and they spend most of their time "playing." They naturally are inclined to explore their environments and to create play situations (see Figs. 3-1 to 3-3). Play is also the most common therapeutic intervention tool used by pediatric occupational therapists.

Many definitions of play have been developed, as well as ways of categorizing play behaviors and skills. However, some basic common elements help define an activity or

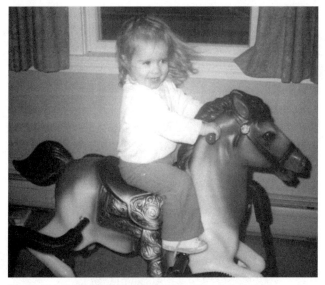

Figure 3-1 Toddler enjoying riding her rocking horse.

occupation as play and distinguish play from other types of occupations or activity (see Bundy, 1997; Brasic-Royeen, 1997; Missiuna and Pollock, 1991; Morrison and Metzger, 2001). These common characteristics of play include the following:

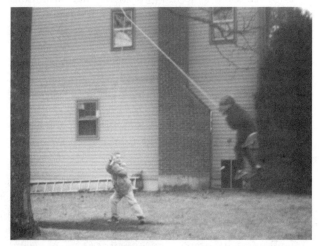

Figure 3-2 Friends creating new ways to swing.

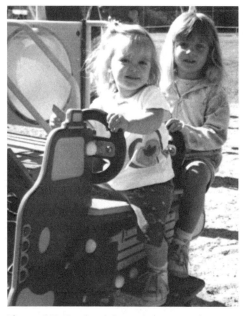

Figure 3-3 Cousins sitting together on a playground riding toy.

- is fun, joyous
- involves doing or participating, whether the play is sedentary (like knitting) or active (like swimming)
- involves free choice, is nonobligatory, and is intrinsically motivating; children always "play" because they want to and never because they have to
- allows the "player" to guide the play situation and is relatively free from rules
- is focused most on the process or the means instead of on the outcome
- often involves pretending or using one's imagination and is not bound by reality

Piaget believed that type of play progressed based on cognitive maturity (cited by Bukatko and Daehler, 2001) (see Figs. 3-4 to 3-6). The first type, **sensorimotor play**, extends into the second year of life and is characterized by the infant's repeated motor movements and the infant's pleasure simply from the experience of seeing, hearing, touching, and holding. The next stage, **sym-**

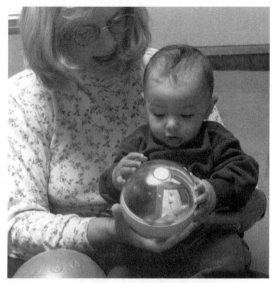

Figure 3-4 This infant, engaged in exploratory, sensorimotor play is very curious. He enjoys looking at and feeling the large ball.

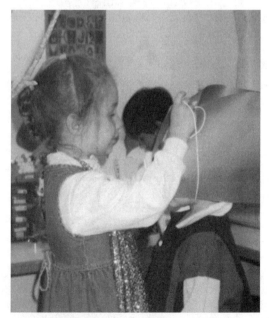

Figure 3-5 Prechoolers, dressing up like kings and queens, are engaged in symbolic play.

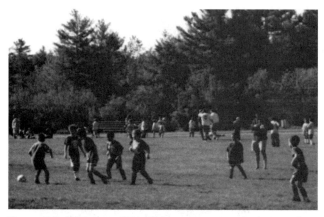

Figure 3-6 Children aged 7 to 9 years play an organized game of soccer, which provides opportunities to learn about cooperation and competition.

bolic play, extends from 2 to 6 years of age, as the child begins to interpret the world in terms of images and symbols and has the capacity to use language and to pretend. A third type of play is games with rules, which typically begins around 5 years of age. This type of **interactive play** is more organized and structured, and it integrates the concepts of cooperation and competition with others.

Another way to categorize and describe play is by the level of social interaction or participation (Knox, 1997). For example, **solitary play** is when a child plays alone. **Parallel play** occurs when children play comfortably next to each other, possibly sharing materials and conversing, but their play agendas and activities are separate. **Social play** involves play activities that are shared and requires children to interact directly with one another during play. Social play involves cooperation, mutually agreed-on roles or rules, social interchange, and (often) competition.

Despite the common characteristics of play described previously, the quantity and quality of play behavior and the reasons for play change as individuals move from infancy to childhood to adulthood. The salient play characteristics typical of children of various ages are described in Table 3-2. From this table, you can see that infants and young children engage in a great deal of exploratory and sensory motor play. Through play, they learn about their

TABLE 3-2	DEVELOPMENT OF PLAY SKILLS
Age	**Typical Play Behaviors and Skills**
0–3 months	Enjoys exploratory and sensorimotor play; explores by reaching for and touching objects; derives pleasure from just seeing, hearing, and feeling; visually tracks objects and loves to look at faces; may become easily overstimulated; alert, attentive play periods are relatively short (10–15 min at a time); may enjoy an infant swing or playing on the floor and in a caregiver's lap; caregiver-infant interactions during play assist in developing attachment behaviors
4–8 months	Enjoys exploratory and sensorimotor play; explores by reaching for, touching, and grasping objects; transfers objects from hand to the other; likes to move arms and legs and often will bring feet to hands when supine; pivots and plays in a sitting position; scoots on tummy; derives pleasure from seeing, hearing, and feeling; grasps, shakes, and throws objects; mouths objects; begins to enjoy simple cause-effect toys such as push buttons, rattles, activity mats, and overhead play gyms (child is supine and reaches over head for hanging toys); plays on floor and in high chair; may coo, squeal, laugh, and communicate through cries and facial expressions; interactive during play primarily with caregivers; notices other children and begins to imitate
9–12 months	Continues with exploratory and sensorimotor play; begins to use toys according to their purpose; play involves more mature manipulation of objects; points, rolls ball, releases toys into container, bangs, throws, and mouths objects; enjoys cause-effect, noisy toys, simple shape sorters, dolls, activity centers, and pop-up toys; crawls or walks to explore the environment; attached to caregivers and may interact briefly with other infants; likes to observe and imitate others
1–2 years	Engages in a lot of gross motor play; enjoys walking fast or running, climbing, riding a kiddy car or other push riding toys and pull toys; runs, jumps, and climbs, often without regard to safety factors; more complex fine motor play develops, and manipulative play involves sorting, inserting large puzzle pieces, stacking, and pulling apart; likes to throw, pound, and dump

(continued)

TABLE 3-2	DEVELOPMENT OF PLAY SKILLS (*Continued*)
Age	**Typical Play Behaviors and Skills**
1–2 years	objects; social play begins to emerge at a very basic level; interested in watching others play; begins limited pretend and social play, but is possessive of toys; tendencies for parallel play; likes all kinds of toys, including dolls and action figures, shape sorters, simple construction toys, riding toys, balls, sensory toys, and pop-up toys; enjoys playground equipment (climbing, sliding, swinging) designed for toddlers; likes looking at picture books with adults and pointing at pictures
2–3 years	With the increase in use of language during this period, the child engages in symbolic and pretend play and begins to shift from parallel play to more interactive forms of play; talks to self during play and begins to use language when playing with others; shows a variety of emotions during play and likes to role-play adult roles; may enjoy action figures, dolls, and other pretend people; may continue to be possessive of toys; likes to imitate; gross motor play includes using playground equipment with some assistance, learning to ride a tricycle, jumping with both feet clearing the ground together, simple ball play (e.g., kicking and tossing a medium-sized ball), and running around, climbing, and dancing; fine motor play includes painting and scribbling; large construction toys and insert puzzles and more complex cause-effect toys that introduce preschool concepts such as colors, shapes, letters, and numbers; continues to be interested in picture books; enjoys sensory play like Play Dough, water, and sand play
3–5 years	Engages in creative and group play, and associative play dominates by 4 years as the child learns to share and take turns and is interested in friends; continues to enjoy role-playing and dressing up, and creating elaborate pretend play situations; may begin to play simple board games, such as checkers or Candyland; with respect to gross motor play, the child becomes proficient on playground equipment, including being able to pump a playground swing; likes to ride a bike with training wheels; may begin to participate in more structured recreational or sports activities, such as swimming, dance, and

(*continued*)

TABLE 3-2	DEVELOPMENT OF PLAY SKILLS (*Continued*)

Age	Typical Play Behaviors and Skills
3–5 years	skiing; enjoys running around, jumping, hopping, climbing, and ball playing; manipulative play skills include painting and coloring, simple drawings, copying basic shapes and some letters, scissor use and simple craft activities, construction toys, and computer play; begins to develop an interest in the finished product of construction play; may become more interested in television and may begin to play videogames
5–7 years	Enjoys games with rules, such as board games, and becomes much more involved in organized sports and recreation in the community; learns specific skills such as swimming, skating, and bike riding or playing a musical instrument, and preferences for certain play activities become more prevalent; plays well with others and enjoys social interaction and play to reach a common goal; understands concepts of cooperation and competition, and the importance of friendships increases; independence during play increases with the extension into neighborhoods and the homes of peers; sedentary play and leisure activities (watching television, reading, and playing computer games or videogames) may also increase
7–11 years	Further development of leisure interests; typical play activities of children this age include participation in organized and recreational sports activities, listening to or playing music, doing craft activities, playing computer games or videogames, watching television and movies, and reading; peer relations and social competencies are important, and leisure time spent with friends increases dramatically; a child's self-identity and self-perceptions are largely influenced by their participation with certain peers and by their interests

(continued)

physical environments and other contexts; experiment with adult roles; develop cognitive, social-emotional, and motor skills; and build meaningful relationships with caregivers, other family members, and friends. Infants, toddlers, and preschool children spend most of their waking hours playing. They need to have ample opportunities to

TABLE 3-2	DEVELOPMENT OF PLAY SKILLS (*Continued*)

Age	**Typical Play Behaviors and Skills**
12–18 years	Further development of leisure interests; typical leisure activities include organized and recreational sports, music, crafts and hobbies, computer use and videogames, television, and movies; adolescents most often make their own decisions regarding their use of leisure time; most leisure time is spent with peers, often just hanging out and talking on the phone, with less time engaging in leisure activities with family members; peer acceptance and peer group norms and values are very influential in how adolescents spend their leisure time

Adapted from Bundy A. Play and playfulness: what to look for. In: Parham LD, Fazio LS, eds. Play in Occupational Therapy. St Louis: Mosby–Year Book Inc, 1997:52–66; Case-Smith J. Development of childhood occupations. In: Case-Smith J, ed. Occupational Therapy for Children. 4th Ed. St Louis: Mosby, 2001:71–94; Knox S. Development and current use of the Knox Preschool Play Scale. In: Parham LD, Fazio LS, eds. Play in Occupational Therapy. St Louis: Mosby–Year Book Inc, 1997:35–51; Morrison C, Metzger P. Play. In: Case-Smith J, ed. Occupational Therapy for Children. 4th Ed. St Louis: Mosby, 2001:528–544; and Sroufe LA, Cooper RG, DeHart GB. Child Development: Its Nature and Course. 2nd Ed. New York: McGraw-Hill, 1992.

access a variety of play materials, to make play choices, and to engage in play with other children as well as adults.

In the elementary school years, play tends to become more structured and social, with the introduction of activities such as organized sports, summer camp programs, and participation in Cub Scouts or Girl Scouts. School-aged children spend more time in group activities than alone or in dyads and show a clear preference for play with same-sex peers (Maccoby and Jacklin, 1987). Sedentary activities such as watching TV, talking with friends, reading, and playing videogames and board games are also common play occupations of school-aged children. Depending on the physical environment, or neighborhood, children older than 5 or 6 years often can venture outside to play with other neighborhood children with limited supervision. They may ride bikes or scooters; organize and play a game of basketball, hide and seek, or street hockey; or just "hang out" (Figs. 3-7 and 3-8). School-aged children get much enjoyment from spending time playing in the homes of their friends or having friends play at their house.

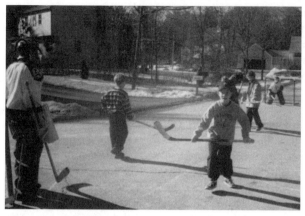

Figure 3-7 A neighborhood game of street hockey. Although this social play has organization and rules, the structure and format were developed by the children.

The amount of time spent in play decreases from the preschool period, with the introduction of school activities and demands and as school-aged children begin to take on more responsibility for completing personal self-care tasks and household chores. Play interests, choices, skills, and expe-

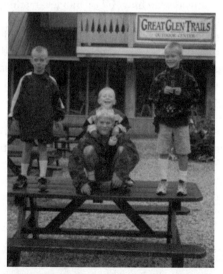

Figure 3-8 Friends just "hanging out." Conversing with friends is one of the most frequent pastimes of older, school-aged children.

riences and "who" a child plays with are important factors that begin to shape a child's self-perception. A child's active engagement in play within their families and communities is also important to foster a sense of belonging, to provide joy, and to help cultivate a child's respect for life.

In the adolescent years, play occupations, sometimes now referred to as **leisure** activities, become more established as the adolescent develops a stronger sense of self and a desire to develop their interests and skills and to belong to a specific peer group. During adolescence, the issues of self-identity, sexuality, and independence are brought to the forefront. Adolescents, for the most part, have much more control over their use of leisure time, and they tend to "play" alongside their peers rather than alone or with family members. They may challenge the scope and domains of parental authority, particularly with respect to the use of their free time.

According to Csikszentmihalyi and Larson (1984), adolescents spend 40% of their time engaged in leisure activity. Most of their leisure time is spent talking with peers, either on the telephone or when just hanging out with friends. Other leisure time is commonly spent participating in competitive or recreational sports activities and games, listening to music, watching TV or movies, reading, doing arts or hobbies, and playing videogames.

The acquisition of **social competencies** is vital for the adolescent to successfully participate in play. In addition to establishing membership in a peer group, adolescents usually have one or two close friends. Intimate relationships also emerge during this period. Several studies have examined the personal qualities that contribute to one's popularity. Qualities that have emerged consistently in the literature include having a pleasing personality, attractiveness, being athletic, being helpful and friendly, conforming to peer norms, being flexible and tolerant, acting naturally and confidently without being conceited, and being the "life of the party" (Gormly and Brodzinsky, 1993).

As adolescents struggle to claim their independence, identities, and social acceptance, their vulnerability toward antisocial or mental health problems increases (Kovacs, 1989). Drug and alcohol abuse, risky sexual behavior, depression, eating disorders, and violence, including gang-related activity, are among the common problems seen in adolescents. Quality family relations, including engagement in some family leisure time, and consistent parenting, characterized by a balance of supervision and rule imposition with freedom, independence, and responsibility, are some factors that may encourage healthy uses of leisure of time.

Participation in Basic and Instrumental Activities of Daily Living, and Vocational Activities

The ability to perform **basic activities of daily living** (bathing, toileting, dressing, eating, and functional mobility) are some of the most important skills children learn as they mature. Not only must children learn to take care of their personal care needs and general health and well-being, but they are required to perform self-care activities in ways that are consistent with societal and cultural norms (see Fig. 3-9). Cultural factors and parenting styles are influential in a child's development of self-care skills and therefore

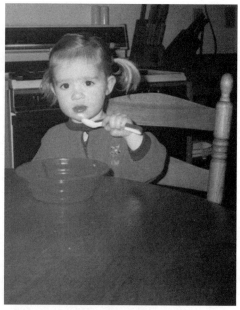

Figure 3-9 This 18-month-old is eating breakfast and is learning how to use a spoon.

need to be considered during your evaluations. Such contextual factors influence when and how a child develops and performs self-care skills, and they play an important role in determining the value that families place on their children's level of independence or competencies with certain skills. The typical progression of skill development in the areas of bathing and grooming, dressing, and toileting are presented in Table 3-3. The development of feeding skills alongside oral motor skills is presented in Table 3-4.

In addition to basic self-care skills, children need to develop **basic home management skills, community living skills,** and some **vocational skills** in preparation for adulthood. Children begin to show an interest in helping others and in participating in household tasks by imitating simple household tasks like wiping the table and vacuuming as early as 2 years of age (Fig. 3-10). Children can help with simple tasks like putting away their toys, wiping spills, and putting dirty clothes in the laundry by 3 to 4 years of age. Providing elementary-aged children with regularly scheduled, simple chores, such as setting the dinner

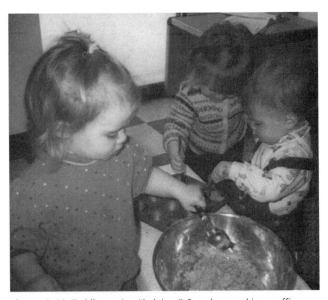

Figure 3-10 Toddlers enjoy "helping." Seen here making muffins, each child is busy helping in his or her own way.

table, emptying the garbage, and tidying up, teaches them responsibility and helps them feel like they are part of a family. Interestingly, girls often participate in household chores more than boys (Seymour, 1988). By the time children are 10 years of age, many can prepare simple meals with supervision, use the telephone appropriately, manage small amounts of money, vacuum, dust, make their bed, and fold clean clothes and put them away.

Contextual factors greatly influence a child's level of skill and participation in household, community living, and vocational activities. Family expectations, needs and priorities, opportunities, and cultural norms all influence the extent to which and the type of skills that are practiced and learned in these areas. For example, large families with limited resources may expect their older children to help more with household chores and may give them child care-giving responsibilities. Some parents may encourage part-time or summer employment outside of the home at an earlier age than others. Peer influences can also positively or negatively influence a child's willingness to participate in such activities, particularly in the adolescent years.

Empirical studies, for the most part, are supportive of adolescent employment, particularly when work experiences are coordinated with school curricula (Gottfredson, 1985). This author suggested that part-time jobs during the high school years help adolescents prepare for adulthood and may decrease dropout rates.

As adolescents prepare to make the **transition from high school** to the workforce or college, one of the most difficult tasks they face is choosing a career or an area of study in college. This is much truer today than ever because of the level of freedom and the large number of available career choices. For adolescents with disabilities, the transition may be more challenging. In addition to vocational activities, transition planning includes determining possible living arrangements and knowledge of the level of supervision or assistance required for community living and participation. Such transition planning for children with disabilities begins before age 16 years, as mandated by special education federal legislation (Individuals With Disabilities Education Act, 1997). Related service providers such as occu-

(*Text continued on page 114*)

TABLE 3-3	DEVELOPMENT OF SELF-HELP SKILLS		
Age	Toileting	Dressing	Bathing and Grooming
1–2 years	Indicates when wet or soiled; indicates need to go to the bathroom by 2 years of age	Cooperates, e.g., pushes arm through sleeve and finds arm hole; removes socks, shoes, and hat; holds leg out to assist in pulling pants on; helps pull down pants	Enjoys bathing; shows some interest in assisting to wash face, hands, and body parts; may resist grooming activities
2–3 years	Develops daytime control with few accidents; goes independently but needs help to wipe self and manage clothing; needs reminders and diapers at night	Removes coat, simple pajamas, and sweatpants; removes socks and shoes; puts on front-button shirt or coat; can unzip and undo large buttons; requires assistance to put on pullover garments like T-shirts	Participates actively in washing self in the tub but requires assistance; can wipe face with cloth and wash hands at the sink with supervision and cues; assists in brushing teeth; may resist grooming activities
3–4 years	Daytime and nighttime control; fully independent except may need help to wipe self and manage clothing fasteners	Can undress upper- and lower-body garments; can put on pullover garments with occasional assistance to orient correctly and straighten; puts on pants except fasteners; can undo and do up large buttons and zip up jacket when the zipper is engaged; puts on shoes and socks except tying bow	Can wash self in the tub with supervision except washing hair; washes hands and face at the sink independently; actively participates in tooth brushing but requires help to do a thorough job; assists with brushing hair; wipes nose; may resist grooming activities

Age			
5–6 years	Fully independent	Independent except with clothing selection and occasional difficult fasteners such as belts and back zippers	Requires supervision only for grooming and tooth brushing, with reminders; bathes self with help to set up water and wash hair and supervision for safety
7–9 years		May begin to select clothing and appropriate clothing for weather	Fully independent in bathing and grooming, although the child may need cues
10+ years		Independent; may begin to assist in purchasing and selecting own clothes; becomes more particular about type and style of clothing	Becomes more interested in appearance and takes more care and interest in grooming activities; may begin to shower daily as early as 9–10 years of age and may apply deodorant; girls develop an interest in makeup in the early teen years

Adapted from Furuno S, O'Reilly KA, Hosaka CM, Inatsuka TT, Allman TA, Zeisloft B. Hawaii Early Learning Profile (HELP). Palo Alto, CA: Vort Corporation, 1984; Orelove F, Sobsey D. Mealtime skills. In: Orelove F, Sobsey D, eds. Educating Children With Multiple Disabilities: A Transdisciplinary Approach. 4th Ed. Baltimore: P.H. Brookes Publishing Co, 1991:335–372; and Shepherd J. Self-care and adaptations for independent living. In: Case-Smith J, ed. Occupational Therapy for Children. 4th Ed. St Louis: Mosby, 2001:489–527.

TABLE 3-4 | DEVELOPMENT OF ORAL-MOTOR AND FEEDING SKILLS

Age	Oral-Motor Skills	Feeding Skills
0–6 months	Has rooting and sucking reflexes; learns to coordinate suck-swallow breathe patterns at 2–4 months; suction on nipple is strong by 4 months	Nursing or bottle-fed formula
6–12 months	Develops strong up and down tongue movements during sucking without any fluid loss; has up and cown munching jaw movements with solid foods, which progresses to some diagonal jaw movements during chewing around 7–8 months; lateral tongue movement develops; rotary chewing develops at approximately 12 months; sitting posture and head and trunk control improve and contribute to ability to self-feed	Continues to drink formula from the bottle or to nurse; learns to hold own bottle at 6–8 months; may drink from sippy cup (cup with lid and spout) around 8 months; begins to eat soft baby foods at 5–7 months; finger feeds self by 7–8 months, including baby cookies; may begin to use spoon by 10–12 months; may transition from bottle to cup at 12 months

1–2 years	Rotary chewing becomes proficient, and the child can manage soft meat and a variety of table foods cut into small pieces; lip closure around cup develops; oral-motor movements become refined as speech develops	Can use a spoon to scoop and feed self, with some spilling; holds cup with lid well and drinks without difficulty; may begin to drink from small cup without a lid at 2 years; tolerates a variety of food textures and eats typical adult foods provided they are cut small enough
2–5 years		Becomes proficient in using a spoon and fork and a cup without a lid, with occasional spilling; manages soup with spoon at 4–5 years
5–10 years		Learns to open food packages and to spread with a knife; cuts meat at 5–8 years; follows table manners

Adapted from Case-Smith J, Humphry R. Feeding intervention. In: Case-Smith J, ed. Occupational Therapy for Children. 4th Ed. St Louis: Mosby, 2001:453–489; Clark. Oral-2motor and feeding issues, #9. AOTA Self Study Series: Classroom Applications for School-Based Practice. Bethesda, MD: American Occupational Therapy Association, 1993; Morris S, Klein M. Pre-feeding skills. Tucson, AZ: Therapy Skill Builders, 1987.

pational therapists play an important role in this process. They may assist in the evaluation of student vocational interests, abilities, and skills; in linking individuals with available community agencies, support networks, and resources; and, most important, in assisting adolescents and their parents identify and fulfill their dreams and priorities related to their child's transition to adulthood.

Participation in School Activities

In the United States as well as most other countries, children are legally required to attend school. Here in the United States, from age 5 or 6 years, children typically spend about 6 hours a day at school, 5 days a week, 10 months of the year (Fig. 3-11). The ultimate aim of formal education is to provide children with the necessary skills to function successfully and independently as responsible and contributing members of society (Bukatko and Daehler, 2001). However, given the amount of time that

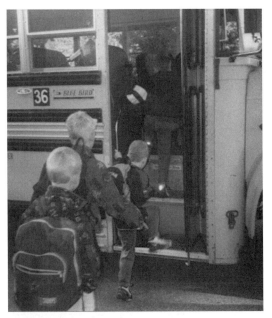

Figure 3-11 Children being picked up for school and riding the school bus.

children spend in school, their school experiences have a profound impact on many aspects of their development, including social and emotional skills, self-concept and self-esteem, and overall psychological well-being.

Special education legislation, as outlined in Chapter 1, mandates and guides the delivery of special education and related services so that all children receive appropriate education programs in the least restrictive environment possible. Whether you work as an occupational therapist in a school setting or another environment, it is essential to include as a part of your evaluations of school-aged children an analysis of the children's abilities to participate in school activities. It is important to find out how the children that are referred to you do in school academically, as well as socially; what they like and dislike about school; and whether they are challenged by any of the curricular and extracurricular school activities that they need or want to do. As with the other areas of occupation, a child's participation and performance in school is influenced by contextual factors, task demand factors, and child factors. Therefore, learning about the child's skills and abilities, academic strengths and challenges, and school activity preferences is important. Equally important is consideration of the child's educational contexts, including physical spaces, seating, his or her teacher's teaching style and the program's educational philosophy, the ratio of adults to children, and the main curricular components and expectations.

Family, Peer, and Community Relationships and Participation

Families play a powerful role in their children's overall development and contribute significantly to a child's resiliency or vulnerabilities in adverse situations (Humphry and Case-Smith, 2001). Family relationships are the most stable or enduring relationships throughout an individual's life, and the family context cannot be separated from a child's development. The concept of "family" today has many definitions, and family constitution or membership varies tremendously within the same culture and across different cultures and ethnic communities.

According to Humphry and Case-Smith (2001), families serve six major functions: (1) providing and fostering affection; (2) providing emotional support; (3) socializing family members for participating in occupations outside the family; (4) providing recreational opportunities; (5) promoting health and independence in basic activities of daily living; and (6) preparing for formal education and employment.

Families are unique not only in membership but in the ways that they construct shared and individual roles, responsibilities, and routines. Viewing the family from a systems or ecological perspective emphasizes the idea that changes in any part of the system (new job for a parent; a new sibling; a sick grandparent) impacts every member of that family system in some way. Regardless of the methods or processes by which families operate, the adults and children go about completing their daily occupations in ways that are perceived to be most efficient and that promote homeostasis. Family functioning is measured by variables such as the amount of time family members spend with one another, their communication and interaction patterns, economic stability, the general physical and emotional health of the family members, stress factors, and internal and external resources.

Understanding what being a family member means for a particular child is essential in your evaluation process. There are many sources of diversity among families, such as the influences of family membership and structure (single parents, grandparents as primary caregivers, same-sex parents, etc.), ethnic and cultural background and traditions, socioeconomic status, parental educational backgrounds and occupations, social support networks (including extended family and friends), and parenting style and practices. These sources of diversity contribute to defining the kinds of roles, responsibilities, and activities that a particular child might be expected to assume or actively participate in as a family member. Children's occupations related to family relationships and participation may involve engaging in leisure, play, and recreational activities with family members, e.g., spending an afternoon on the family boat or playing a traditional touch football game on Thanksgiving Day. Other important family activities might include sitting quietly during Sunday church services, baby-sitting younger siblings, eating and conversing together during mealtimes, watching television with siblings, going through a bedtime routine, and doing assigned household chores.

A child's ability to establish and maintain healthy relationships with family members is equally, if not more, important as his or her ability to participate in family activities and in fulfilling one's role as a family member. As noted earlier, family relationships provide stability, nurturance, and emotional support not only throughout childhood but for a lifetime. As families raise their children through the stages of early childhood, middle childhood, and adolescence, family members must adapt to developmental changes that affect the nature of their relationships with one another and the type of family routines, rituals, tasks, and activities experienced by family members.

Although peers, the media, and teachers all play a significant role in a child's socialization, parents probably have the greatest influence on the development of a child's personality, values, and future behaviors. In infancy, parents focus on caregiving activities, nurturance, and helping the child feel safe and secure and on developing healthy attachment behaviors. During the preschool years, parents focus more on teaching basic self-care skills, such as dressing and toileting, and begin to make more deliberate efforts to promote their child's socialization. Parents of preschoolers have the challenging task of helping their children regulate their emotions, exhibit self-control, and learn cultural and social norms, morals, and values. During early and middle childhood, the focus of parents shifts to helping their children succeed at school, although parents continue to help their children develop self-control and peer relations and learn sociocultural norms and values. During this time they may encourage certain extracurricular activities, such as sports activities, regularly invite their children's friends over to play etc., all of which influence a child's peer relations and network. Finally, in adolescence, parents encourage their children to develop independence and responsibility and to exercise value-based decision making (Bukatko and Daehler, 2001).

There is an abundance of literature studying the relationships between mothers and their children and fathers and their children and among siblings and the ways in which such relationships influence child development (Bukatko and Daehler, 2001; Patterson and Blum, 1996). During your evaluations of children, it is important to consider the nature of the relationships among family members and how such relationships may be contributing to a child's vulnerabilities or resiliency and overall development.

The family system may be viewed as a subset of a larger **ecosystem**. Ecological models consider broader contextual factors such as economic and political climates and community resources, all of which influence family functioning and community participation. It is important for children and their families to feel like they are part of a community. Communities provide recreational and social opportunities, and they support the general health and well-being of family systems. Community participation as an occupation for children may include various activities, such as going to the mall with family or friends, attending church services, playing with children in the neighborhood, doing volunteer work, using recreational facilities, and participating in recreational programs. Self-maintenance activities, such as accessing medical services, shopping for groceries, and going out for meals, are also considered an aspect of community participation. Community participation involves both family activities and activities with peers. It is important to realize that every community is unique in the quality and quantity of resources it provides and in the ease with which families can access the resources and programs that are available. All children and their families need to feel like they belong, and "sense of belonging" is enhanced through time spent engaged in activities in their communities.

In addition to family and community participation, **peer relationships** are considered an important occupation of childhood. Older school-aged children and adolescents often report that they have the most fun when with their peers, regardless of the activities that they do together. Besides simply experiencing pleasure, friendships provide a context for the development of social skills, self-esteem, and a child's identity. Good peer relations have also been associated with academic success and have been shown to decrease the risk for deviant or problem behaviors later in life (Crick and Ladd, 1993).

The nature and importance of peer relationships and of friendships change throughout the various stages of development. Infants and young toddlers are interested in peers, and they observe and may explore one another, but actual interactions are brief and rarely involve mutual exchanges of behavior. During the preschool years, children engage in all types of play with peers, with a tendency to prefer play with children of the same sex. During this period, peer interactions provide a rich context for development in many domains, such as social-emotional, language, motor, and cognition. Peers provide both models and reinforcers for learning about social norms and for the development of social competence.

In the elementary years, children begin to select playmates that have similar behavioral styles and skills, and peers are especially important in the development of feelings of self-worth and to validate and share interests. School-aged children often play in large groups and may single out one or two more special playmates with whom they spend greater amounts of time. During adolescence, peer relationships become more intense, with intimate friendships developing. It is common for middle school children and young teenagers to form cliques or to be identified with a specific crowd. Friendships during this time provide a source of support and leisure and recreational opportunities. Peer pressure, positive and negative, can be influential in the behavior of children, particularly from the seventh to the twelfth grade (Berndt, 1999). As adolescents near adulthood and become more confident with who they are, they begin to worry less about being accepted into groups and are more interested in developing relationships with individuals of the same sex and the opposite sex. Nonetheless, establishing friendships, feeling accepted by peers, and having opportunities to share, learn, and have fun with peers is important for every child throughout their development.

THE DEVELOPMENT OF MOTOR SKILLS

The development of motor skills and capacities experienced by infants and children influences the ways in which children engage in developmentally appropriate tasks and activities. Sensorimotor behavior supports their learning and for infants and toddlers is the primary way that they communicate to us what they know or want. The motor skills and behaviors discussed in the following subsections—reflexes, automatic reactions and postural control, and fine motor, gross motor, and oral-motor skills—represent many of the child factors included in the AOTA's Practice Framework.

Reflexes

Sensorimotor development in early infancy is largely characterized by reflexes that dominate infant movement and behavior. Reflex behavior is an important survival function for the infant and is primarily controlled by the more primitive central nervous system areas, including the spinal cord and brainstem levels (Mathiowetz and Haugen, 1995). For example, the infant's crying behavior signals a need for care, and the rooting reflex helps the infant locate food. As the infant develops, these primitive reflexes gradually disappear, most by the first year of life. Many of the reflexes are incorporated into more complex, voluntary actions. For example, the grasp reflex (with pressure into the palm of the hand, the infant curls the fingers inward and grabs onto the finger or object) predominates until the infant is about 3 or 4 months of age. By 4 or 5 months of age, the infant can voluntarily reach out, and he or she learns to grab desired objects.

It is important to examine reflex behavior in infants and children with suspected neurologic impairments because these reflex behaviors serve as a little window into the child's central nervous system. Because data are available that describe these reflexes and identify when they tend to emerge and disappear, they serve as soft signs of neurodevelopmental maturation (Farber, 1991; Mathiowetz and Haugen, 1995). The examination of reflex behavior is also important because persistence of these reflexes sometimes negatively influence a child's ability to perform functional motor skills. For example, if the grasp reflex persists, the child will experience difficulty in developing hand use. Asymmetries in the performance of reflexes may also indicate a pathologic condition. Therefore, understanding the influence of primitive reflex patterns on behavior helps explain "why" an infant or child may be experiencing difficulty and is an indicator of neurodevelopmental maturation. The most common reflexes and when they emerge and disappear are presented in Table 3-5.

Automatic Reactions and Postural Control

Automatic or postural reactions, including righting, protective, and equilibrium reactions, develop as the child begins to gain postural control for functional movement. Although these reactions typically are automatically performed in response to a stimulus, we can exert some level of control over them. Most of these automatic reactions are controlled at the midbrain level of the central nervous system (Mathiowetz and Haugen, 1995). The development of these reactions has been reported to occur first in prone, then in supine, then in sitting, then in a quadruped (crawling/hands and knees) position, and, finally, in standing (Nichols, 2001). They primarily serve as mechanisms for maintaining our balance as we move or are moved. As with the primitive reflexes, automatic reactions provide information about the quality of a child's movement, may be influential in a child's ability to acquire increasingly complex motor skills, and provide information about neurodevelopmental maturation. The developmental progression of automatic reactions is detailed in Table 3-6.

The development of postural control for movement requires the ability to move against gravity and proximal stability (Nichols, 2001; Gilfoyle et al., 1990). Typical positions assumed by infants and children as they gain motor control and stability in supine, prone, sitting, quadruped (crawling position), and standing and major gross motor milestones in the first year of life are presented in Table 3-7. Figures 3-12

(*Text continued on page 129*)

TABLE 3-5 | PRIMITIVE REFLEX PATTERNS

iReflex	Stimulus	Response	Age Reflex Emerges	Age Reflex Fades
Rooting	Stroke side of mouth	Head turns toward stimulus	28 weeks' gestation	3–7 months (longer in nursed babies)
Sucking	Place finger on lips	Infant sucks	28 weeks' gestation	3–7 months
Palmar grasp	Pressure with a finger into palm of the hand	Fingers flex in a tight grip	30 weeks' gestation	3–4 months
Placing (arms)	Touch back of hand on tabletop	Places hand on table with flexion then extension	36 weeks' gestation	2 months
Placing (legs)	Touch top of foot on tabletop	Places foot on table with flexion then extension	36 weeks' gestation	2 months
Stepping	Upright, slightly tip forward, placing some weight on bottom of feet	Rhythmic, alternating steps	35 weeks' gestation	3 months
Plantar grasp	Pressure with a finger on the bottom of each foot	Toes flex	25 weeks' gestation	12 months

Asymmetrical tonic neck	In supine, turn head to one side	Extension of arm and leg on face side; flexion of limbs on skull side	1 month	4 months
Tonic labyrinthine	Observe posture in prone; observe posture in supine	Primarily a flexed posture in prone and an extension posture in supine	40 weeks' gestation	3 months
Symmetrical tonic neck	Prone over lap, flex neck, observe; extend neck, observe	With neck flexion, arms flex and legs extend; with neck extension, arms extend and legs flex	4 months	10 months
Landau	Hold in prone suspension	Neck, arms, and legs extend	5 months	7–18 months
Moro	Support in semireclined position, release support momentarily	Arms abduct and extend and externally rotate, followed by flexion and adduction	28 weeks' gestation	4 months

Adapted from Mathiowetz V, Haugen JB. Evaluation of motor behavior: traditional and contemporary views. In: Trombly CA, ed. Occupational Therapy for Physical Dysfunction. 4th Ed. Baltimore: Williams & Wilkins, 1995:157–185; and Gilfoyle E, Grady A, Moore J. Children Adapt. 2nd Ed. New York: Slack Inc, 1990.

TABLE 3-6 | THE DEVELOPMENT OF AUTOMATIC REACTIONS

Reaction	Stimulus	Response	Age Response Emerges
Protective responses	In sitting, gently push the child off balance, to the front, to each side, and backwards	Arm extends and places on the supporting surface to prevent falling	Front, 6–7 months; side, 7–10 months; back, 9–12 months
Head righting	In sitting or in vertical suspension, tilt the child gently from side to side and front to back	Child moves head position in opposite direction to maintain the head in alignment with the body	3–4 months
Neck on body righting	In supine, rotate the child's head to one side	Body rotates and child rolls over to prone either as a unit (log roll) or segmentally, with some dissociation of the upper and lower body	Segmental rolling emerges at 4–5 months
Body on body on righting	In supine, rotate the child's hips to one side	The child rotates upper body and rolls over to align the body	Segmental rolling emerges at 4–5 months

| Equilibrium reactions | Can be tested with the child facing you, in prone, supine, quadruped, and standing; tilt the child's supporting surface to one side, then the other side | When tilted to child's left, lateral flexion of the right side of the trunk, head righting, abduction and extension of the right arm and leg, and trunk rotation to the right; when tilted to the right, lateral flexion of the left side of trunk, abduction and extension of the left arm and leg, trunk rotation to the left, and head righting | Prone, 5–6 months; supine, 7–8 months; sitting, 7–10 months; quadruped, 9–12 months; standing, 12–20 months |

Adapted from Mathiowetz V, Haugen JB. Evaluation of motor behavior: traditional and contemporary views. In: Trombly CA, ed. Occupational Therapy for Physical Dysfunction. 4th Ed. Baltimore: Williams & Wilkins, 1995: 157–185; Gilfoyle E, Grady A, Moore J. Children Adapt. 2nd Ed. New York: Slack Inc, 1990; and Nichols D. Postural control. In: Case-Smith J, ed. Occupational Therapy for Children. 4th Ed. St Louis: Mosby, 2000:266–288.

TABLE 3-7	DEVELOPMENT OF GROSS MOTOR SKILLS DURING THE FIRST YEAR		
Age	**Skills in Prone and Supine**	**Skills in Sitting and Quadruped**	**Standing and Mobility**
2–4 months	In prone, lifts head 90° and weight bears mainly through the lower chest and forearms; in supine, keeps head in midline; when pulled into sitting by the hands from supine, may begin to flex the neck to keep the head aligned with the shoulders around 4 months	Unable to sit unsupported; has a rounded back in sitting, with occasional back extensor activity	Stepping reflex elicited when held in standing
4–6 months	In prone, props on hands with back and neck extension, weight shifts from upper to lower trunk and from side to side; in supine, brings feet to mouth, shifts weight laterally, and moves into sidelying	May begin to sit independently for short periods, with hand support forward and side; may begin to move in and out of sitting around 6 months	Rolls prone to supine and supine to prone; pivots in prone; partial weight bearing in supported standing
6–8 months	No longer likes to play for extended periods in prone or supine	Sits well independently with back fully extended; can use both hands in play when sitting; may begin to crawl or scoot forward; moves in and out of sitting easily	Fully weight bearing in supported standing; may take some steps with both hands held

| 8–10 months | | Crawls well | Pulls self up to stand using furniture; walks with one or both hands held |
| 10–12 months | | | May take first steps; walks well with one hand held or behind a push toy |

Adapted from Gilfoyle E, Grady A, Moore J. Children Adapt. 2nd Ed. New York: Slack Inc, 1990; Nichols D. Postural control. In: Case-Smith J, ed. Occupational Therapy for Children. 4th Ed. St Louis: Mosby, 2001:266–288; and Folio R, Fewell R. Peabody Developmental Motor Scales–2. 2nd Ed. Austin, TX: Pro-Ed, 2000.

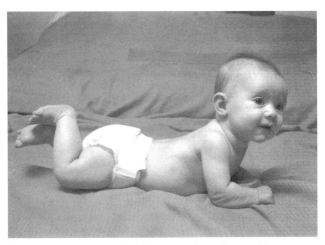

Figure 3-12 This 4-month-old infant can lift up her head in prone, and she seems comfortable in this position. She cannot pivot or scoot forward, and she weight bears through her mid to upper chest and forearms. Her hands tend to be in a fisted position, and she kicks her legs spontaneously.

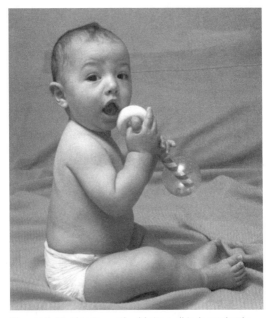

Figure 3-13 This 8-month-old sits well independently with his back straight and can free his hands for play.

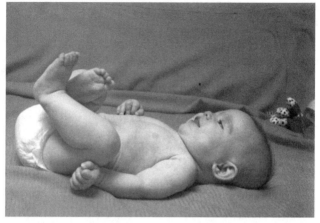

Figure 3-14 In supine, this 4-month-old lifts her feet up, but she cannot lift her buttocks off of the floor. She moves her hands freely, brings them to midline, and can keep her head in midline.

to 3-14 provide examples of postural control and stability observations that can be made of infants in prone, supine, and sitting positions, and more formal clinical observations are described in Chapter 5.

The evaluation of some reflexes, automatic reactions, and postural control is included in standardized assessment tools such as the Motor Assessment of Infants (Chandler et al., 1980) and the Toddler and Infant Motor Evaluation (Miller and Roid, 1994). Quality of movement, reflexes, automatic reactions, and postural control characteristics may also be examined through formal and informal clinical observations of the infant or child as he or she moves through and maintains various positions if you have a good understanding of what to look for. For example, it is necessary to know the stimulus or position necessary to elicit a certain reflex or response and what motor or behavioral responses are expected for infants and children of various ages.

The ability to execute normal automatic reactions, the integration of primitive reflexes, and the development of postural control provide a foundation for the development of fine and gross motor skills. If a child's fine or gross motor skills are delayed or if a child experiences difficulty learning or executing certain motor skills, then an evaluation of these foundational motor components may be helpful in uncovering some of the reasons why the difficulties exist.

The Development of Gross, Fine, and Oral-Motor Skills

Our ability to learn and perform motor skills depends on various underlying neuromotor and musculoskeletal factors (the AOTA's uniform terminology [1994] [Appendix F] and Practice Framework [Appendix A]), including muscle strength, postural control and balance, muscle tone, range of motion and agility, motor coordination, and motor planning. Sensory awareness and processing, particularly of the tactile, proprioceptive, and visual sensory systems, also contributes to motor skill performance. Cognitive components, such as attention and problem-solving abilities, and psychological components, such as motivational factors, interests, and values, may be contributing factors. Contextual factors, such as a lack of experience with certain motor activities, may also affect a child's level of competency in performing certain motor tasks. Play, the primary occupation of children, is greatly affected by a child's ability to move accurately and efficiently around his or her environment and to access and manipulate objects. Typical progression of gross motor skills is presented in Tables 3-7 to 3-9.

The ability to learn and perform fine motor skills depends on various component skills, including reach, grasp, release, dexterity and in-hand manipulation, bilateral hand use, and visual-motor skills (Exner, 2001; Case-Smith, 1996). Therefore, when conducting comprehensive evaluations of fine motor skills, all of these areas should be examined. The normal developmental progression of fine motor components is presented in Tables 3-10 and 3-11. Various typical motor sequential patterns contribute to our ability to acquire increasingly complex fine motor skills over time (Exner, 2001). Generally, upper-extremity function progresses from gross to fine, proximal to distal, mass to specific, ulnar to radial, and more asymmetrical patterns to symmetrical patterns.

The development of oral-motor skills is necessary for both feeding and expressive language. Because the oral-motor movements (particularly tongue movements) involved in producing language are very intricate, oral-motor performance may be viewed as a type of fine motor skill. Speech pathologists are specifically trained in the analysis of oral-motor movements for speech production and swallowing, and their roles overlap with occupational therapists in the evaluation of oral-motor function. The development of oral-motor and feeding skills is presented in Table 3-4.

COGNITIVE DEVELOPMENT

Cognitive development refers to development of the mental processes of thinking and understanding and the ability to use the senses to gather information and make sense of the world. The development of cognitive skills is a complex process that begins as soon as the infant is born, or even earlier, and has largely been studied by developmental psychologists. Several theorists have proposed explanations for how cognitive development takes place. Jean Piaget is probably the best-known theorist, and he developed a series of stages describing cognitive development from infancy to young adulthood (Piaget, 1971). Some specific cognitive skills expected of children at various ages are presented in Table 3-12.

Communication and Language Development

The development of language is largely considered a cognitive skill; however, expressive language does require the motor planning, sequencing, and coordination of intricate oral motor movements. Infants communicate primarily through crying behavior, and parents report that they can determine their child's basic needs (tired/need for sleep and hunger) through their child's cries within the first 3 months of life (Sroufe et al., 1992). Research evidence also supports the idea that infants are preprogrammed or genetically predisposed to attend to language (Sroufe et al., 1992). By 3 to

TABLE 3-8 | DEVELOPMENT OF GROSS MOTOR SKILLS FROM 1–5 YEARS OF AGE

Age	Functional Mobility	Gross Motor Skills
1–1.5 years	Walks well for very short distances; may use a wide base of support, and falls frequently, especially over uneven ground; uses high chair for meals, crib for sleeping, and stroller for long walks	Crawls up and down stairs with supervision; rides a push riding toy; throws toys with little accuracy, climbs up a ladder with supervision
1.5–2 years	Begins to run, although poorly coordinated; jumps down from a raised surface of a few inches with one foot leading; walks short distances; typically uses stroller for longer walks; continues to use high chair for meals and crib for sleeping	Jumps clearing both feet from the ground; walks up and down stairs by placing both feet on each step and using the railing for support; kicks and tosses a ball but with little accuracy; uses a playground slide with minimal assistance and enjoys playing on playground equipment designed for toddlers; likes to walk with pull toys, and operates push riding toys easily
2–3 years	Begins to negotiate playground equipment but needs close supervision; needs assistance to use standard-sized toilets; continues to require a stroller for longer walks; running is better coordinated, and can stop and change direction without falling; climbs in and out of car seat and out of crib	Learns to ride a tricycle; enjoys playground equipment and likes to run, jump, and climb; jumps down from a raised surface with both feet together; catches a medium-sized playground ball against chest; stands on one foot for a few seconds and may learn to hop

3–5 years	Manages sitting and mobility skills safely to use standard toilet and to get in and out of child's bed; may use a booster seat for meals; often does not use stroller after 4 years of age except for longer walks; manages stairs going up and down with alternate feet by 4–5 years	Begins to learn specific skills such as swimming and skating; may participate in organized recreational programs such as soccer, dance, or swimming lesson s; can pump a playground swing and play safely on playground equipment by 4–5 years; gallops and skips; rides a two-wheeled bike with training wheels; turns a somersault and hops on one foot; can toss, kick, and catch a medium-sized ball with some degree of accuracy

Adapted from Case-Smith J. Development of childhood occupations. In: Case-Smith J, ed. Occupational Therapy for Children. 4th Ed. St Louis: Mosby, 2001:71–94; Gilfoyle E, Grady A, Moore J. Children Adapt. 2nd Ed. New York: Slack Inc, 1990; Nichols D. Postural control. In: Case-Smith J, ed. Occupational Therapy for Children. 4th Ed. St Louis: Mosby, 2001:266–288; Folio R, Fewell R. Peabody Developmental Motor Scales–2. 2nd Ed. Austin, TX: Pro-Ed, 2000; and Sroufe LA, Cooper RG, DeHart GB. Child Development: Its Nature and Course. 2nd Ed. New York: McGraw-Hill, 1992.

TABLE 3-9	DEVELOPMENT OF GROSS MOTOR SKILLS FROM 5–18 YEARS OF AGE

Age	Gross Motor Skills
5–7 years	Rides a two-wheeled bike without training wheels; learns specific skills, such as skating and swimming; begins to participate in organized team and individual sports activities; can complete complex, multistep motor sequences, such as those required for dance or martial arts; participates in regular physical education programs at school
7–12 years	Can run longer distances with good endurance; throws a small ball toward a target, and can catch a small ball; may participate in more advanced competitive sports activities; develops specific interests and skills related to gross motor recreational activities; begins to concern self with physical fitness, and participates in regular physical education programs at school
12–18 years	Continues to concern self with physical fitness and to participate in regular physical education programs at school; participation in team sports may decline during this period; some adolescents will advance their skills in specific sports activities, and participation in sports and physical recreational activities is influenced by sociocultural factors, family and peer influences, and individual preferences

Adapted from Case-Smith J. Development of childhood occupations. In: Case-Smith J, ed. Occupational Therapy for Children. 4th Ed. St Louis: Mosby, 2001:71–94; Folio R, Fewell R. Peabody Developmental Motor Scales–2. 2nd Ed. Austin, TX: Pro-Ed, 2000; Sroufe LA, Cooper RG, DeHart GB. Child Development: Its Nature and Course. 2nd Ed. New York: McGraw-Hill, 1992; and Bukatko D, Daehler M. Child Development: A Thematic Approach. Boston: Houghton Mifflin Co, 2001.

4 months of age, the infant learns to smile and use facial expressions to communicate surprise, distress, or happiness. At this time, they also engage in prelanguage cooing and babbling. Between 6 and 12 months of age, infants develop the use of gestures, such as pointing toward desired objects, waving bye-bye, and lifting up their arms to communicate that they want to be picked up (Acredolo and Goodwyn, 1988).

Infants learn and use their first words, such as "mama, juice, ball, or dada," by the end of their first year. Between

(*Text continued on page 139*)

TABLE 3-10	DEVELOPMENT OF REACH, GRASP, AND RELEASE OF OBJECTS

Age	Description of Typical Patterns Used
0–2 months	Palmar grasp reflex is strong; hands are usually fisted; has visual regard for hands; puts hands in mouth; unable to reach
2–4 months	Palmar grasp reflex is strong; hands often fisted and clasped together; begins to reach for objects, with poor motor control; holds onto objects placed in hands momentarily with gross fisted grasp; often puts hands in mouth; frequent visual regard for hands; demonstrates full active range of movement of fingers, wrists, and hands during spontaneous play, but unable to grasp objects
4–8 months	Palmar grasp reflex weakens; reaches for objects easily; picks up and holds objects like a 1" block using primarily an ulnar, palmar, fisted grasp; shakes rattles; picks up tiny objects with a raking motion and by trapping the object between the thumb and the side of the index finger (scissor grasp); holds larger objects (e.g., a tennis ball) using both hands together, with poor control; transfers objects from one hand to the other; proficient at bringing hands to mouth; puts objects in mouth
8–12 months	Palmar grasp reflex fades; uses gross fisted grasp on objects using the radial side of the hand more than the ulnar; uses a mature pincer grasp to pick up tiny objects; transfers objects from one hand to the other; uses both hands together to pick up and hold larger objects (e.g., a tennis ball or a baby bottle); has voluntary release of objects, although poorly controlled, and likes to throw, bang, and dump objects; does not yet demonstrate a hand preference; does not have in-hand manipulative abilities
1–2 years	Uses a mature pincer grasp to hold tiny objects (object held between the tip or pad of the index finger and the thumb, with the thumb opposed and the wrist extended); uses a radial palmar grasp to pick up a 1" cube and a pronated finger grasp on cylindrical objects; has controlled release of objects; stacks about five 1" blocks; scribbles when given a crayon

Adapted from Case-Smith J. Development of childhood occupations. In: Case-Smith J, ed. Occupational Therapy for Children. 4th Ed. St Louis: Mosby, 2001:71–94; Gilfoyle E, Grady A, Moore J. Children Adapt. 2nd Ed. New York: Slack Inc, 1990; Exner CE. Development of hand skills. In: Case-Smith J, ed. Occupational Therapy for Children. 4th Ed. St Louis: Mosby, 2000:289–329; Folio R, Fewell R. Peabody Developmental Motor Scales–2. 2nd Ed. Austin, TX: Pro-Ed, 2000; and Sroufe LA, Cooper RG, DeHart GB. Child Development: Its Nature and Course. 2nd Ed. New York: McGraw-Hill, 1992.

TABLE 3-11	DEVELOPMENT OF FINE MOTOR DEXTERITY, IN-HAND MANIPULATION, AND BILATERAL HAND USE

Age	Characteristics
2–4 months	Holds onto objects placed in hands momentarily with gross fisted grasp; hands often clasped together
4–8 months	Shakes rattles; picks up tiny objects with a raking motion and by trapping the object between the thumb and the side of the index finger (scissor grasp); uses both hands together to hold larger objects (e.g., a tennis ball or a baby bottle), but with poor control; begins to transfer objects from one hand to the other; proficient at bringing hands to mouth; puts objects in mouth
8–12 months	Transfers objects from one hand to the other easily; uses both hands together to pick up and hold objects such as a tennis ball and a baby bottle; has voluntary release of objects, although poorly controlled, and likes to throw, bang, and dump objects; does not demonstrate a hand preference; able to pick up tiny objects with a pincer grasp; finger feeds self; does not have in-hand manipulative abilities
1–2 years	Beginning in-hand manipulation (able to move objects from fingers into palm or to perform finger to palm translocation); has controlled release of objects and can play with shape sorter toys and large insert puzzles; stacks about three to five 1" blocks; uses both hands together to carry objects and claps hands; will stabilize with one hand while manipulating with the other; can scribble; uses a spoon and drinks from a sippy cup; tosses a small ball, with little accuracy; activates more complex cause-effect push-button toys and pop-up toys; turns pages of a book and likes to point isolating index finger; enjoys banging and throwing objects
2–3 years	In-hand manipulation develops and can move objects from the palm into the fingers without help from the other hand (palm to finger translocation); develops controlled release with shoulder, elbow, and wrist stability; stacks about four to seven 1" blocks; uses both hands together to open simple containers with lids; winds wind-up toys; strings large beads; copies a simple line and a circle; colors large forms; snips with scissors

(continued)

TABLE 3-11	DEVELOPMENT OF FINE MOTOR DEXTERITY, IN-HAND MANIPULATION, AND BILATERAL HAND USE (*Continued*)

Age	Characteristics
3–4 years	Can do simple fasteners such as large buttons and uses hands well to dress and undress; uses mature tripod grasp on a pencil, colors in the lines, and copies simple shapes; strings beads; cuts out large shapes with scissors; builds with construction toys such as Tinker Toys and Duplo blocks; dresses dolls
4–6 years	Learns to tie shoes; learns to print name; copies all letters, numbers, and short sentences; can do fasteners such as buttons, snaps, and zippers; begins to use fork and knife for cutting; completes puzzles up to 20 pieces; enjoys building with construction toys such as Lego blocks; opens most packaging; manages a computer mouse
7–10 years	Learns cursive writing; develops good dexterity for constructing models and other craft projects with small pieces; puts together intricate Lego and other types of models; can create craft projects using tools such as hole punches, staplers, glue, scissors, and needle and thread; can tie knots, cut small shapes with scissors, and make intricate life drawings; proficient and graceful with eating utensils; can manage more complex hygiene activities, such as using nail clippers and styling hair; uses computer keyboard and mouse, although does not use proper keyboarding technique for typing; may develop a specialized skill, such as playing the piano or needlework
10+ years	Typing speed and ability to manage motor skills for computer use increase; further develop drawing and handwriting abilities; may develop specific fine motor skills depending on interests, such as pursuing various forms of art and music; develops tool use for completing school science projects and activities in courses such as woodworking and home economics

Adapted from Case-Smith J. Development of childhood occupations. In: Case-Smith J, ed. Occupational Therapy for Children. 4th Ed. St Louis: Mosby, 2001:71–94; Gilfoyle E, Grady A, Moore J. Children Adapt. 2nd Ed. New York: Slack Inc, 1990; Exner CE. Development of hand skills. In: Case-Smith J, ed. Occupational Therapy for Children. 4th Ed. St Louis: Mosby, 2000:289–329; Folio R, Fewell R. Peabody Developmental Motor Scales–2. 2nd Ed. Austin, TX: Pro-Ed, 2000; and Sroufe LA, Cooper RG, DeHart GB. Child Development: Its Nature and Course. 2nd Ed. New York: McGraw-Hill, 1992.

TABLE 3-12	DEVELOPMENT OF COGNITIVE SKILLS

Age	Cognitive Skills
0–6 months	Infant learns to repeat behaviors that produce desired results (sucking thumb, shaking rattle); very interested in his or her environment, especially faces; increases time being awake, alert, and attentive; mouths objects; recognizes familiar caregivers; has a basic understanding of simple cause-effect; coos and babbles
6–12 months	Infant learns to coordinate schemes applied to external objects to accomplish a goal, e.g., uses a stick to retrieve a toy; imitates simple motor movements and sounds; recognizes his or her name; begins to use tools, such as spoons, for intended purpose; begins to understand that objects exist even if they cannot be seen (beginning object permanence) by searching for hidden objects; simple problem solving through trial and error; figures out simple shape sorters, pop-up toys, etc.; likes peek-a-boo; responds to simple requests
1–2 years	Develops a mature concept of object permanence (searches for hidden objects even when the child does not see the object be moved); experiments and plays with objects in novel ways; evidence of memory functions (knows where favorite toys are kept, uses words, plays strange with unfamiliar adults); proficient in activating cause-effect toys; groups and stacks toys; develops the capacity for representation or the ability to use ideas or images to represent objects or events, allowing language to emerge
2–4 years	Develops basic preschool skills, such as identifying name, body parts, age, colors, shapes, and some letters and numbers; counts objects up to 10 and may rote count further; discovers causal mechanisms, such as winding up a toy; performs meaningful actions in a sequence, such as carrying out a pretend tea party; speaks in small sentences
4–6 years	Develops an understanding of conservation of liquid volume; understands that the same amounts can appear different depending on the size and shape of the container; develops number concepts to allow for simple addition and subtraction problems; may begin to read simple words; concepts of time develop, including telling time and knowing days of the week

(continued)

TABLE 3-12	DEVELOPMENT OF COGNITIVE SKILLS (*Continued*)
Age	**Cognitive Skills**
6–12 years	Academic performance in reading, writing, and mathematics becomes important; reading should be proficient by the end of third grade; begins abstract thinking, with logical reasoning; understands consequences of actions
12+ years	Ability for advanced abstract reasoning develops, and more advanced academics, and more responsibility for self-directed learning; has knowledge of major current events; understands consequences, and logical reasoning is more advanced and can project into the future

Adapted from Case-Smith J. Development of childhood occupations. In: Case-Smith J, ed. Occupational Therapy for Children. 4th Ed. St Louis: Mosby, 2001:71–94; Furuno S, O'Reilly KA, Hosaka CM., Inatsuka TT, Allman TA, Zeisloft B. Hawaii Early Learning Profile (HELP). Palo Alto, CA: Vort Corporation, 1984; Gormly A, Brodzinsky D. Lifespan Human Development. 5th Ed. Fort Worth: Harcourt Brace Jovanovich Publishers, 1993; Piaget J. Psychology and Epistemology: Towards a Theory of Knowledge. New York: The Viking Press, 1971; Sroufe LA, Cooper RG, DeHart GB. Child Development: Its Nature and Course. 2nd Ed. New York: McGraw-Hill, 1992; and Thomasgard M, Shonkoff JP. Mental retardation. In: Zeanah CH, ed. Handbook of Infant Mental Health. 5th Ed. New York: Guilford Press, 1993:250–259.

2 and 3 years of age, the use of language increases dramatically, with the average 3-year-old using 3,000 to 4,000 words (Miller, 1981) and constructing three- to five-word phrases or short sentences. Language is typically well developed by 4 years of age (Sroufe et al., 1992).

SOCIAL AND EMOTIONAL DEVELOPMENT AND BEHAVIOR

During the first 3 months of life, infant behavior is largely reflexive and to some extent preprogrammed with built-in protective mechanisms (Sroufe et al., 1992). These predispositions assist the infant in developing self-regulation and play an important role in allowing the infant to get his or her physiological and psychological needs met. They also provide a foundation for healthy social-emotional growth. Infant cries may be distinguished to signal hunger, need for sleep, or desire for attention. Infants are believed to be pre-programmed to be attracted to human faces because of the type of contrasting visual stimuli provided by faces and to respond to human speech. Brazelton and Cramer (1990) report that infants are also adaptable in that they can accommodate, to some extent, to the style of caregiving provided by their parents or caregivers.

Reciprocity refers to mutual social exchanges between the infant and caregiver, and this behavior becomes more evident as the infant's awake time increases; as motor behavior, including reaching and head control, improves; and as the infant becomes more able to attend. By the end of the third month of life, most infants begin to show some preferential responsiveness to their parents or caregivers and begin to smile. Social exchanges/reciprocity also increases as the infant becomes more responsive and able to display feelings of frustration, surprise, sadness, and happiness through facial expressions and vocalizations. It is important that infants experience some consistency and routine in their care; that they feel loved, safe, and secure; and that they are well-nourished.

In understanding typical infants, it is important to consider temperament. Temperament refers to various behavioral dimensions, including general mood, activity level, adaptability, persistence, and emotional responsiveness (Rothbart and Bates, 1998). Research indicates that individual differences with respect to these behavioral characteristics (e.g., a fussy versus an easy-going baby or a shy versus an outgoing infant) are relatively stable or consistent over time and may reflect the child's individual personality traits (Rothbart, 1989). It is important for parents to understand their infant's temperament because it is often helpful for them to adjust their parenting style to better match the temperament of their child.

Attachment is defined as an enduring emotional bond between infant and caregiver (Bowlby, 1982). Attachment relationships are crucial because they become part of the infant's coping skills (they look for comfort specifically from their caregiver when stressed) and they provide the infant with feelings of security necessary for the child to later explore the environment freely (Ainsworth et al., 1978). Various behaviors have been identified to evaluate attachment behavior in infants. For example, typically by 10 to 12 months of age, infants display separation anxiety or feelings of distress when separated from their parent or primary caregiver. At this age, infants show emotion when reunited with their caregiver (who left temporarily), such as squealing and bouncing up and down, with arms outstretched. Different patterns of attachment have been described by Ainsworth et al. (1978), and an abundance of literature has examined the relationships between caregiving and parenting qualities and attachment behavior (Dewolff and van Ijzendoorn, 1997).

Toddlers, from about 1 to 3 years of age, learn to cope with rules while becoming more self-reliant and further develop their social skills and relationships with family members and peers. As they develop language, they become interested in interacting with others. Toddlers decrease the amount of physical closeness or contact with their caregivers and begin to show less distress when a caregiver temporarily leaves. Toddlers are interested in objects in their environment and like to ask about and share their experiences with others and imitate. They begin to engage in social, interactive play with peers by 3 years of age, begin to take turns, and can perform different roles in games such as hide-and-seek. During the toddler period, knowledge of one's own existence as a separate individual emerges, so the development of self-concept begins.

The daunting task of parents during this period is to encourage their toddler's growth and independence while setting limits and clear expectations for appropriate behavior. It is believed that the child's ability to adapt during this period is largely the result of the quality of early attachment relationships as well as the consistency and clarity of parental guidance at this time (Frankel and Bates, 1990). Some specific behaviors reflective of healthy infant and toddler psychosocial and emotional development are presented in Table 3-13.

During the early and middle childhood years, children become increasingly more self-reliant. By age 5 years, many play in their neighborhoods or at a friend's house, and most attend kindergarten. Peer relationships and the development of early relationships become increasingly important. Social competency is difficult to measure, but some indicators include number of friends, ability to get along with others, being liked by peers, and teacher ratings of social competency (Sroufe et al., 1992). Social competency is important because not only is being with friends fun but peer groups provide a rich learning environment

TABLE 3-13	PSYCHOSOCIAL AND EMOTIONAL DEVELOPMENT OF INFANTS AND TODDLERS
Age	**Description of Typical Behavior**
0–3 months	Communicates through cries, facial expressions, and body postures; turns in the direction of voices and establishes eye contact; enjoys physical contact; is calmed by sucking, being held; begins to smile
3–6 months	Expresses emotions such as happiness, sadness, anger, fear, or distress; interested in faces; is calmed when picked up; smiles, coos, babbles, and laughs; explores body parts visually and through touch and mouthing; looks in response to name; develops strategies to calm self; establishes a routine for eating and sleeping; may begin to distinguish caregiver from others
6–12 months	Imitates sounds and may speak first words; plays strange by being distressed when caregiver leaves; anticipates being picked up by reaching; loves to explore environment; displays likes and dislikes; enjoys watching others and is interested in other children; enjoys social games with adults, e.g., patty-cake; waves bye-bye and responds appropriately to facial expressions; may begin to show distress when caregiver leaves around 9–10 months
1–2 years	Displays clingy behavior with the parent and is often distressed when the parent leaves but moves freely away from the parent when the parent is nearby; likes to do things for self and may resist adult control; enjoys being the center of attention, recognizes familiar people versus strangers; identifies self in mirror; shows toy preferences; expresses a variety of emotions; expresses affection, including giving hugs and kisses; may display anger and frustration with temper outbursts; language use increases; identifies familiar objects, including body parts and animals; has a vocabulary of at least 15–20 words and follows simple directions, such as "bring me your shoes"; interacts briefly with other children but engages mostly in solitary and parallel play

(continued)

TABLE 3-13	PSYCHOSOCIAL AND EMOTIONAL DEVELOPMENT OF INFANTS AND TODDLERS (Continued)
Age	**Description of Typical Behavior**
2–3 years	Has good receptive language; vocabulary is >500 words; engages in simple dialog with sentences of 3–5 words; defends possessions but begins to learn to share and take turns, although difficult for the child; begins to socially interact in play and likes to be with peers; is shy with strangers; can follow simple rules; may display anger and frustration with temper outbursts; takes pride in achievements; insists on performing self-care tasks independently

Adapted from Bates E, Bretherton I, Snyder L. From First Words to Grammar. Cambridge, England: Cambridge University Press, 1988; Bloom L. Language acquisition in its developmental context. In: Damon W, series ed; Kuhn D, volume ed. Handbook of Child Psychology: Volume 2: Cognition, Perception, and Language. 5th Ed. New York: Wiley, 1998:309–370; Bukatko D, Daehler M. Child Development: A Thematic Approach. Boston: Houghton Mifflin Co, 2001; Furuno S, O'Reilly KA, Hosaka CM, Inatsuka TT, Allman TA, Zeisloft B. Hawaii Early Learning Profile (HELP). Palo Alto, CA: Vort Corporation, 1984; Case-Smith J. Development of childhood occupations. In: Case-Smith J, ed. Occupational Therapy for Children. 4th Ed. St Louis: Mosby, 2001:71–94; and Sroufe LA, Cooper RG, DeHart GB. Child Development: Its Nature and Course. 2nd Ed. New York: McGraw-Hill, 1992.

for children. Peer groups provide opportunities for children to learn about social and cultural norms and values and the concepts of fairness and right from wrong.

As children reach school age, they learn to take more responsibility for self-control, monitoring and directing their own behavior. Children learn to wait, to develop some tolerance for frustration, and to control their anger. They also develop empathy and learn to value helping others. Their sense of self continues to develop through their experiences and as their unique strengths, challenges, and interests become more apparent. They also become more aware of gender and gender differences. Generally, most school-aged children have positive self-esteem and self-evaluate their behaviors and skills favorably. They begin to compare their abilities with those of their peers at around 7 years of age (Ruble, 1983).

The increasing importance of peers, however, does not lessen the developmental importance of the family on the child's social-emotional growth during this period. Family

TABLE 3-14	PSYCHOSOCIAL AND EMOTIONAL DEVELOPMENT OF SCHOOL-AGED CHILDREN AND ADOLESCENTS

Age	**Typical Social Behaviors, Emotional Development, and Self-Concept**
4–6 years	Plays well with others, shares, and takes turns; has and enjoys being with friends; can visit at a friend's house and may sleep over at a friend's house for the first time; follows simple rules and directions; apologizes for errors that hurt others; likes to help others and shows empathy; displays and can identify various emotions in self; has some self-control over anger or disappointment when denied own way; views self positively and views self with respect to physical traits; takes pride in own work and construction play; timid/shy with strangers; has definite likes and dislikes
6–12 years	Peer relationships are important, and more time is spent with peers than with family members; loyal friendships develop; school-aged children view themselves in terms of psychological traits by comparing themselves with others and through peer group membership; gender roles become more pronounced; develop self-discipline and self-control and respect for persons in authority
12+ years	Adolescence may be a time of emotional turmoil, as they experience puberty and struggle with their desire for independence but need for support, guidance, and limit setting; adolescents may engage in risk-taking behavior, and they continue to be greatly influenced by their peer group; early adolescence is often characterized by a struggle with self-identity, moodiness, and a tendency to return to immature behavior when stressed. By the final high school years, adolescents demonstrate more emotional stability, self-reliance, and concern for the future; a decrease in conflict with parents; and an increased capacity for delayed gratification and compromise. Some signs of psychosocial and behavioral problems include a marked decline in school performance, anxiety, hyperactivity and sleep and eating disturbances; persistent noncompliance and aggressive behavior, excessive complaints of physical ailments, opposition to authority figures, withdrawn behavior, negative self-statements and depressed mood, difficulties with social relationships, and substance abuse

Adapted from American Academy of Child and Adolescent Psychiatry. Facts for Families: Being Prepared: Know When to Seek Help for Your Child. Available at: http://www.aacap.org/publications/factsfam/,1997; American Academy of Child and Adolescent Psychiatry. Facts for Families: Normal Adolescent Development: Late High School Years. Washington DC, Available at: http://www.aaacap.org/factsfam/.1997; Cronin A. Psychosocial and emotional domains. In: Case-Smith J, ed. Occupational Therapy for Children. 4th Ed. St Louis: Mosby, 2000:413–452; and Sroufe LA, Cooper RG, DeHart GB. Child Development: Its Nature and Course. 2nd Ed. New York: McGraw-Hill, 1992.

relationships change as the child matures and is given more responsibility. Various types of parenting styles, from permissive to strict, have an impact on children's behavior. However, regardless of parenting style, support from caregivers, their interest and involvement in their children's activities, and their guidance and approval are all important to every child's growing sense of self and ability to adhere to social norms and responsibilities. Some specific behaviors reflective of typical psychosocial and emotional development during the early and middle childhood years are described in Table 3-14.

As discussed previously, adolescence is a time of transition, as teenagers struggle to claim their independence, their identities, and social acceptance. During this time, vulnerability toward antisocial or mental health problems such as substance abuse, gang-related violence, and depression increases (American Academy of Child and Adolescent Psychiatry, 1997b,c). Peer relations are very important, as is their sense of self, self-confidence, and perceived competencies. Some of the important psychosocial issues and competencies facing adolescents are included in Table 3-14.

SUMMARY

This chapter provides a brief overview of some of the more common theories of development and basic developmental principles. Important theoretical concepts related to occupational therapy were also presented, along with information about the common occupations of childhood. Finally, the normal progression of skill acquisition in a variety of developmental domains was provided. This information is provided as background to assist you during the evaluation planning process. The age-specific activities, occupations, and skill areas discussed will give you some idea of what to expect of children at various ages. This information will help you focus your evaluation on the most important child competencies and contextual factors when evaluating children of various ages and will help you interpret your evaluation data.

References

Acredolo, L.P., & Goodwyn, S.W. (1988). Symbolic gesturing in normal infants. *Child Development, 59*, 450–466.

American Academy of Child and Adolescent Psychiatry (1997a). Facts for Families: Being prepared: Know when to seek help for your child. Washington, DC. Available at http://www.aacap.org/publications/factsfam/.

American Academy of Child and Adolescent Psychiatry (1997b). Facts for Families: Normal Adolescent Development: middle and early high school years. Washington, DC. Available at www.aacap.org/publications/factsfam/.

American Academy of Child and Adolescent Psychiatry (1997c). Facts for Families: Normal Adolescent Development: Late high school years. Washington DC, Available at www.aacap.org/publications/factsfam/.

Ainsworth, M., Blehar, M., Waters, E., & Wall, S. (1978). *Patterns of attachment*. Hillsdale, NJ: Erikbaum.

American Occupational Therapy Association (1994). Uniform terminology for occupational therapy- third edition. *American Journal of Occupational Therapy, 49*, 1029–1031.

Angoff, W. (1988). The nature-nurture debate, aptitude and group differences. *American Psychologist, 43*, 713–720.

Bandura, A. (1977). *Self-efficacy: Toward a unifying theory of behavior change. Psychological Review, 84*, 191–215.

Bates, E., Bretherton, I., & Snyder, L. (1988). *From first words to grammar*. Cambridge, UK: Cambridge University Press.

Bayley (1993). *Bayley scales of infant development (BSID-II)*. San Antonio, TX: Psychological Corp.

Berndt, T.J. (1999). Friends' influence on school adjustment. In W. A. Collins & B. Laursen (Eds.), *Minnesota symposia on child psychology: Volume 30, relationships as developmental context* (pp. 85–107). Mahwah, NJ: Erlbaum.

Bloom, L. (1998). Language acquisition in its developmental context. In W. Damon (Series Ed.) & D. Kuhn (Vol. Ed.), *Handbook of child psychology: Volume 2: Cognition, perception, and language* (5th ed., pp. 309–370). New York, NY: Wiley.

Bowlby, J. (1982). *Attachment and loss* (2nd ed.). New York, NY: Basic Books.

Brasic-Royeen, C. (1997). Play as occupation and as an indicator of health. In B. Chandler's (Ed.), *The essence of play*. Bethesda, MD: American Occupational Therapy Association.

Brazelton, T.B., & Cramer, B. (1990). *The earliest relationship*. Reading, MA: Addison Wesley.

Bronfenbrenner, U., & Ceci, S.J. (1994). Nature-nurture reconceptualized in a developmental perspective: Bioecological model. *Psychological Review, 101*, 568–586.

Bundy, A. (1997). Play and playfulness: What to look for. In L.D. Parham & L.S. Fazio (Eds.), *Play in occupational therapy* (pp. 52–66). St. Louis, MO: Mosby–Year Book, Inc.

Butkatko, D., & Daehler, M. (2001). *Child development: A thematic approach.* Boston, MA: Houghton Mifflin Co.

Case, R. (1995). *Intellectual development: Birth to adulthood.* Orlando, FL: Academic Press.

Case-Smith, J. (1996). Fine motor outcomes in preschool children who receive occupational therapy services. *American Journal of Occupational Therapy, 50(1)*, 52–61.

Case-Smith, J. (2001). Development of childhood occupations. In J. Case-Smith (Ed.), Occupational therapy for children (4th ed., pp. 71–94). St. Louis, MO: Mosby–Year Book, Inc.

Case Smith, J., & Humphry, R. (2001). Feeding intervention. In J. Case-Smith (Ed.), Occupational therapy for children (4th ed., pp. 453–489). St. Louis, MO: Mosby–Year Book, Inc.

Chandlers, L., Andrews, M., & Swanson, M. (1980). *Movement assessment for infants, manual.* Rolling Bay, WA.

Christiansen, C., & Baum, C. (1997). *Occupational theory: Enabling function and well-being.* Thorofare, NJ: Slack.

Clark, G. (1993). *Oral-motor and feeding issues, No. 9. AOTA self study series: Classroom applications for school-based practice.* Bethesda, MD: American Occupational Therapy Association.

Crick, N.R., & Ladd, G.W. (1993). Children's perceptions of their peer experiences: Attributions, loneliness, social anxiety, and social avoidance. *Developmental Psychology, 29*, 244–254.

Cronin, A. (2000). Psychosocial and emotional domains. In J. Case-Smith (Ed.), Occupational therapy for children (4th ed., pp. 413–452). St. Louis, MO: Mosby–Year Book, Inc.

Csikszentmihalyi, M., & Larson, R. (1984). *Being adolescent.* New York: Basic Books.

DeWolff, M.S., & van Ijzendoorn, M.H. (1997). Sensitivity and attachment: A meta-analysis of parental antecedents of attachment. *Child Development, 68*, 571–591.

Dunn, W., Brown, C., & McGuigan, A. (1994). The ecology of human performance: A framework for considering the effect of context. *American Journal of Occupational Therapy, 48*, 595–607.

Erikson, E. (1963). *Childhood and society* (2nd ed.). New York: Norton.

Exner, C.E. (2000). Development of hand skills. In J. Case-Smith (Ed.), Occupational therapy for children (4th ed., pp. 289–329). St. Louis, MO: Mosby–Year Book, Inc.

Freud, S. (1966). *Standard edition of the psychological works of Sigmund Freud.* London: Hogarth.

Farber, S.D. (1991). Neuromotor dimensions of performance. In C. Christiansen & C. Baum (Eds.), Occupational therapy. *Overcoming human performance deficits* (pp. 259–282). Thorofare, NJ: Slack Inc.

Flavell, J.H. (1996). Piaget's legacy. *Psychological Science, 7,* 200–203.

Folio, R., & Fewell, R. (2000). *Peabody developmental motor scales–2,* (2nd ed.). Austin, TX: Pro-Ed.

Frankel, K.A., & Bates, J.E. (1990). Mother-toddler problem solving: Antecedents in attachment, home behavior, and temperament. *Child Development, 61,* 810–819.

Furuno, S., O'Reilly, K.A., Hosaka, C. M., Inatsuka, T. T., Allman, T. A., & Zeisloft, B. (1984). *Hawaii early learning profile (HELP).* Palo Alto, CA: Vort Corporation.

Gewirtz, J.L., & Pelaez-Nogueras, M. (1992). B.F. Skinner's legacy to human infant behavior and development. *American Psychologist, 47,* 1411–1422.

Gilfoyle, E., Grady, A., & Moore, J. (1990). *Children adapt* (2nd ed.). New York, NY: Slack, Inc.

Gormly, A., & Brodzinsky, D. (1993). *Lifespan human development* (5th ed.). Fort Worth, TX: Harcourt Brace Jovanovich Publishers.

Gottfredson, D. (1985). Youth employment, crime, and schooling: A longitudinal study of a national sample. *Developmental Psychology, 21,* 419–432.

Hall, C.S., & Lindzey, G. (1978). *Theories of personality development* (3rd ed.), New York, NY: John Wiley.

Humphry, R., & Case-Smith, J. (2001). Working with families. In J. Case-Smith (Ed.), Occupational therapy for children (4th ed., pp. 95–136). St. Louis, MO: Mosby–Year Book, Inc.

Individuals with Disabilities Education Act (IDEA) Amendments of 1997 (PL.105-17). U.S.C. 1400.

Kielhofner, G. (1995). *A model of human occupation: Theory and application* (2nd ed.), Baltimore: Williams & Wilkins.

Knox, S. (1997). Development and current use of the Knox preschool play scale. In L.D. Parham & L.S. Fazio (Eds.), *Play in occupational therapy* (pp. 35–51), St. Louis, MO: Mosby–Year Book Inc.

Kovacs, M. (1989). Affective disorders in children and adolescents. *American Psychologist, 44,* 209–215.

Krantz, M. (1994). *Child development: Risk and opportunity.* Belmont, CA: Wadsworth.

Law, M., Cooper, B., Stewart, D., Rigby, P., & Letts, L. (1996). The person-environment–occupation model: A transactive approach to occupational performance. *Canadian Journal of Occupational Therapy, 63(1),* 9–23.

Maccoby, E.E., & Jacklin, C.N. (1987). Gender segregation in childhood. In R.W. Reese (Ed.), *Advances in child development and behavior (Vol. 20)*. Orlando, FL: Academic Press.

Massaro, D.W., & Cowan, N. (1993). Information processing models: Microscopes of mind. In L.W. Porter & M.R. Rosenweig (Eds.), *Annual Review of Psychology, 34*, 383–425.

Mathiowetz, V., & Haugen, J. B. (1995). Evaluation of motor behavior: Traditional and contemporary views. In C. A. Trombly (Ed.), *Occupational therapy for physical dysfunction* (4th ed., pp. 157–185). Baltimore: Williams & Wilkins.

Miller , G.A. (1981). *Language and speech*. San Francisco, CA: Freeman.

Miller, L.J., & Roid, G.H. (1994). *The T.I.M.E. Toddler and infant motor evaluation: A standardized assessment*. Tucson, AZ: Therapy Skill Builders.

Missiuna, C., & Pollock, N. (1991). Play deprivation in children with physical disabilities: The role of the occupational therapist in preventing secondary disability. *American Journal of Occupational Therapy, 45*, 882–888.

Morris, S., & Klein, M. (1987). *Pre-feeding skills*. Tucson, AZ: Therapy Skill Builders.

Morrison, C., & Metzger, P. (2001). Play. In J. Case-Smith (Ed.), *Occupational therapy for children* (4th ed., pp. 528–544), St. Louis, MO: Mosby–Year Book, Inc.

Nichols, D. (2001). Postural control. In J. Case-Smith (Ed.), Occupational therapy for children (4th ed., pp. 266–288), St. Louis, MO: Mosby–Year Book, Inc.

Orelove, F. & Sobsey, D. (1991). Mealtime Skills. In F. Orelove & D. Sobsey (Eds.), Educating children with multiple disabilities: A transdisciplinary approach, (4th ed., pp. 335–372), Baltimore, M. D.: P.H. Brookes.

Patterson, J.M., & Blum, R.W. (1996). Risk and resilience among children and youth with disabilities. *Archives of Pediatric Adolescent Medicine, 150*, 692–698.

Piaget, J. (1971). *Psychology and Epistemology: Towards a theory of knowledge*. New York, NY: The Viking Press.

Rothbart, M. (1989). Temperament I childhood: A framework. In G. Kohnstamm, J. Bates, & M. Rothbart (Eds)., Temperament in childhood (pp. 59–73), New York, NY: Wiley.

Rothbart, M.K., & Bates, J.E. (1998). Temperament. In W. Damon (Series Ed.) & N. Eisenbereg (Vol. Ed.), *Handbook of child psychology (Vol. 3). Social emotional and personality development* (5th ed., pp. 105–176). New York, NY: Wiley.

Ruble, D. (1983). The development of social comparison processes and their role in achievement-related self-socialization. In T.

Higgins, D. Ruble, and W. Hartup (Eds.), *Social cognitive development*. Cambridge: Cambridge University Press.

Schmidt, R.A. (1988). *Motor control and learning: A behavioral emphasis*. Champaign, IL: Human Kinetics.

Seigler, R. (1983a). Information processing approaches to development. In P.H. Mussen (Ed.), *Handbook of childhood psychology (Vol. 1): History, theory and methods*. New York, NY: Wiley.

Seigler, R. (1983b). Five generalizations about cognitive development. *American Psychologist, 38,* 263–277.

Seymour, S. (1988). Expressions of responsibility among Indian children: Some precursors of adult status and sex roles. *Ethos, 17(4),* 355–370.

Shepherd, J. (2001). Self-care and adaptations for independent living. In J. Case-Smith (Ed.), Occupational therapy for children (4th ed., pp. 489–527), St. Louis, MO: Mosby–Year Book, Inc.

Skinner, B.F. (1957). *Verbal behavior*. New York, NY: Appleton-Century-Crofts.

Sroufe, L.A., Cooper, R.G., & DeHart, G.B. (1992). Child development. Its nature and course (2nd Ed.). US: McGraw-Hill.

Thomasgard, M., & Shonkoff, J.P. (1993). Mental retardation. In C. H. Zeanah's (Ed.), *Handbook of infant mental health* (5th ed., pp. 250–259), New York: Guilford Press.

Vygotsky, L.S. (1978). *Mind in society: The development of higher psychological processes*. Cambridge, MA: Harvard University Press.

Waters, E., & Sroufe, L.A. (1983). A developmental perspective on competence. *Developmental Review, 3,* 79–97.

4

STANDARDIZED ASSESSMENT TOOLS

INTRODUCTION

This chapter provides information about the use of standardized assessment tools. The content is applicable to other occupational therapy practice areas, as most occupational therapy evaluations include the administration of standardized tests. **Norm-** and **criterion-referenced** standardized tools are described. Methods for evaluating **psychometric properties** of tests are presented, and information to help you understand, interpret, and present **standardized test scores** is covered in detail. The chapter concludes with sample reviews of two standardized assessment tools commonly used in pediatrics and tables listing some of the available assessments organized by the skills or content areas measured by each.

DESCRIPTION OF STANDARDIZED ASSESSMENT TOOLS

Standardized assessment tools are those that have specific procedures for administration and scoring. Test materials and forms typically are provided in a test kit, along with a test manual. **Test manuals** describe in detail the purpose(s) of the test and the population for which it was designed. The test construction process should also be described, along with the results of research studies examining the reliability and validity of the tool. Administration and scoring procedures are described in detail so that all individuals trained in its administration and scoring procedures administer the assessment to their clients precisely in the same manner.

Standardized assessment tools are important for providing objective data about client performance. These data may be used for (1) diagnostic purposes; (2) determining the nature and extent or severity of difficulties; (3) evaluating and documenting change in performance over time, such as progress; (4) qualifying an individual for a particular program or service; (5) predicting performance in a related task or future function; (6) program planning purposes; and (7) research purposes. Standardized assessment tools are important for advancing the scientific body of knowledge of professions and for enhancing communication across disciplines. Objective measurement in occupational therapy clinics and for use in applied research will also assist in improving the status of our profession and promote evidence-based practice. There are two types of standardized assessment tools or tests norm referenced and criterion referenced.

Norm-Referenced Assessments

Norm-referenced assessment tools provide scores that are compared with the scores of children from a specific sample, or normative group. Because a child's score on a norm-referenced test is converted to a standard score that is derived from the normative data, the score depends on the average performance of children in the normative group. Norm-referenced assessment tools have detailed information about the normative data in the test manual. It is important that characteristics of the normative group are relevant for your client. For example, norms of children from Denver, Colorado, may not be relevant for children living in rural Alaska; a test of gross motor skills normed on typical children may not be relevant to detect changes in gross motor performance of children with Down's syndrome; or norms of children 9 years of age may not be relevant for children 10 or 11 years of age. Norm-referenced tests typically evaluate a broad array of skills and are particularly good for diagnostic and research purposes, to evaluate change in performance, and to examine the extent or severity of identified delays or dysfunction (Campbell, 1989; Gilfoyle, 1981). Depending on the particular test, norm-referenced tests may or may not be useful for the development of intervention programs.

Criterion-Referenced Assessments

Criterion-referenced assessment tools typically use a rating system or level of mastery to score a child's performance in particular activities, sequential tasks, or skills. This type of test helps describe specifically the skills a child can or cannot do and compares a child's performance with a set of criteria instead of with the performance of others (Montgomery and Connolly, 1987). Criterion-referenced tests may also provide information regarding the amount of help or the methods children use to complete a particular activity. The progression or sequence of skills that a child performs is most important as opposed to the age levels. Some assessment tools, such as the Peabody Developmental Motor Scales–2 (Folio and Fewell, 2000) and the Pediatric Evaluation of Disability Inventory (Haley et al., 1992), are both criterion-referenced and norm-referenced. The former rates the child's abilities on various fine and gross motor skills, and then the child's scores are compared with those from the appropriate normative group (based on age). The test kit also provides activity cards that can be used for intervention purposes.

MAKING THE DECISION TO USE A STANDARDIZED ASSESSMENT TOOL

Your decision to use a particular standardized assessment tool should be made after consideration of several factors, including (1) the specific purpose or areas measured by the test; (2) whether the tool was designed for your client's age and abilities; (3) its psychometric properties,

---

BOX 4-1   QUESTIONS TO AID YOU IN DECIDING WHETHER
              TO ADMINISTER A SPECIFIC STANDARDIZED TEST

What assessment information do you need?

Will the test yield the kind of information you and your clients are looking for?

Are there more efficient means of gathering the same information?

Is the purpose of the test consistent with your guiding frames of reference and the philosophy of your practice and setting?

Will the child be able to tolerate and follow the administration procedures?

What is your competency level in administering the test?

Is the necessary space and equipment available?

How reliable and valid is the test for the situation in which you would like to use it?

What tests have been administered in the past, and what were the results?

---

including the normative data, reliability, and validity (discussed further later in this chapter); and (4) pragmatic factors such as length of time needed, your competency in its administration, space requirements, and cost. Sound **clinical reasoning** will assist you in determining whether the child's results on the test will provide you with the information you are looking for efficiently and whether child characteristics such as attention span and motor, sensory, and cognitive abilities will permit you to administer the test in the standardized way in which it was intended to be administered. A list of questions you may want to ask yourself to help you decide whether to administer a specific assessment tool is provided in Box 4.1. Many standardized pediatric assessment tools have been designed to measure various aspects of performance and skills. Tables 4-1 through 4-6 provide a sample of the tools more commonly used by occupational therapists, organized by the following categories: (1) developmental evaluation and screening tools; (2) tools measuring activities of daily living, functional skills, and play; (3) assessments of sensory motor skills, including gross and fine motor skills, postural control, sensory processing, and

Text continues on page 166

TABLE 4-1 STANDARDIZED DEVELOPMENTAL SCREENINGS AND EVALUATIONS

Test Name (Author[s])	Age Range	Purpose/Domains/Description and General Comments
Denver II (Frankenburg and Dodds, 1992)	0–6 years	A screening tool designed for children at risk for developmental problems. Domains include personal-social, fine motor adaptive, language, and gross motor. Takes 20–30 min to administer; easy to learn; psychometrics are adequate, although the number of test items is relatively small.
Infant-Toddler Developmental Assessment (Provence et al., 1995)	Birth to 36 months	A comprehensive, multidisciplinary, standardized assessment system that uses naturalistic observation and parent report regarding eight developmental domains: gross and fine motor, cognition, language/communication, self-help skills, psychosocial, and emotional. Reliability and validity are adequate; designed to promote early intervention programming.
Miller Assessment for Preschoolers (Miller, 1988)	2 years, 9 months to 5 years, 8 months	Norm-referenced test measuring foundational sensory and motor abilities, including tactile processing and kinesthesia, balance, coordination, and motor planning functions. Also includes some cognitive and language items; has strong psychometric properties; although it was originally designed as a screening tool, further research has supported it as an evaluation tool.
Hawaii Early Learning Profile (Furuno et al., 1984)	0–36 months	A criterion-referenced assessment tool that provides age levels. Domains include personal/social, cognition, communication, self-help, gross motor, fine motor, and visual-motor; a relatively quick and easy screening tool often used by interdisciplinary early intervention teams.

(continued)

TABLE 4-1 | STANDARDIZED DEVELOPMENTAL SCREENINGS AND EVALUATIONS *(Continued)*

Test Name (Author[s])	Age Range	Purpose/Domains/Description and General Comments
The First Step (Miller, 1993)	Preschool children	A norm-referenced screening tool designed to identify preschool children at risk for developmental problems. Domains include cognition, communication, motor, social-emotional, and adaptive behavior. Has strong psychometrics; quick to administer; training is recommended.
Battelle Developmental Inventory (Newborg et al., 1988)	0–8 years	Norm-referenced test including five domains: personal/social, adaptive including self-help skills; motor, expressive and receptive communication, and cognition; information is gathered through structured observations, administration of test items, and interviews and can take 1–2 hours; normative data is strong, and reliability and validity is adequate.
Gesell Preschool Test (Bates-Ames et al., 1980)	2.5–6 years	Norm-referenced test consisting of 13 tests measuring motor, adaptive, language, and personal/social areas. Specialized training is not required, although it does require a fair amount of training and practice to be familiar with the test items. Research on reliability and validity is limited.
Bayley Scales of Infant Development (Bayley, 1993) (also has a screening tool)	1–42 months	Norm-referenced tests, including a mental scale (cognitive, language, personal/social), a psychomotor scale (fine and gross motor skills, sensory integration, quality of movement), and a behavior scale (social, interests, activity level). Takes 45–60 min to administer; strong psychometrics and well researched; training is recommended.

TABLE 4-2 STANDARDIZED ASSESSMENTS MEASURING FUNCTIONAL SKILLS AND PLAY

Test Name (Author[s])	Age Range	Main Purpose(s)
Pediatric Evaluation of Disability Inventory (Haley et al., 1992)	6 months to 7.5 years	Assesses self-care, functional mobility, and social functioning through structured interview, observation, or both. Considers level of caregiver assistance and use of adapted devices; psychometric properties are strong (see review in this chapter).
School Function Assessment (Coster et al., 1998)	Children in kindergarten through sixth grade	Criterion-referenced tool for evaluating child performance, level of participation, and need for assistance in school activities, including both physical and cognitive/behavioral tasks; psychometric properties are strong.
Assessment of Motor and Process Skills (Fisher, 1999); School version (Fisher and Bryze, 1997)	Adults, adolescents, and older children; also a school version	The child is asked to perform five to six tasks from a list of 56 calibrated ADL tasks. The tool measures both process and motor skills, as they relate to task performance; provides information about how the child is performing in a given context; and is used to predict performance in ADL areas. Extensive training is required; psychometrics are strong.
Vineland Adaptive Behavior Scales (Sparrow et al., 1984)	Birth through 18 years	Measures communication, daily living skills, socialization, and motor skills; uses a behavior rating scale that is completed through a structured parent interview; easy to administer; psychometrics are adequate.
Canadian Occupational Performance Measure (Law et al., 1998)	Children of all ages; parents may complete on child's behalf for younger children	Measures the child's performance and satisfaction in areas of self-care, leisure, and productivity through interview. Helpful in prioritizing intervention goals and measuring functional outcomes; well researched, and psychometrics are adequate.

(continued)

TABLE 4-2 | STANDARDIZED ASSESSMENTS MEASURING FUNCTIONAL SKILLS AND PLAY (Continued)

Test Name (Author[s])	Age Range	Main Purpose(s)
Self-Assessment of Occupational Functioning (Henry et al., 1999)	Child version and adolescent-adult version	Self-report measure to be completed during a structured interview. Based on the Model of Human Occupation, it addresses strengths and weaknesses related to volition, habituation, performance, and environment.
Functional Independence Measure (Hamilton and Granger, 1991)	Child version is for children 6 months to 6 years	Universal tool designed to measure rehabilitation outcomes related to functional skills, including self-care, mobility, sphincter control, communication, and social cognition; well researched.
Klein-Bell ADL Scale (Klein and Bell, 1982)	All ages (except infants and toddlers)	Rating scale that measures six areas of function through caregiver and client report or observations. Domains include dressing, elimination, mobility, bathing and grooming, eating, and emergency telephone communication. Research is limited.
Test of Playfulness (Bundy, 1997)	Children of all ages	60-item observational tool that examines criteria for playfulness including intrinsic motivation, suspension of reality, and internal locus of control, in the context of free play; training is required; research is ongoing, and preliminary studies support it as a valid and reliable tool.
Knox Preschool Scales–Revised, (Knox, 1997)	Birth to 3 years	A rating scale for evaluating play behaviors that include space management, including gross motor play behaviors, materials management, pretense-symbolic play, and social participation. Research is limited for this revised edition.
Symbolic Play Checklist (Westby, 1980)	9 months to 5 years	A norm-referenced test designed to assess a child's cognitive and language behaviors through a play observation. A description of 10 stages of play is provided. Research is limited.

ADLs, activities of daily living.

TABLE 4-3 STANDARDIZED TESTS OF SENSORY MOTOR FUNCTIONS, INCLUDING GROSS AND FINE MOTOR SKILLS, POSTURAL CONTROL, SENSORY PROCESSING, AND SENSORY INTEGRATION

Test Name (Author[s])	Age Range	Purpose/Domains/Description and General Comments
Alberta Infant Motor Scale (Piper and Darrah, 1994)	0–18 months	Norm-referenced tool measuring gross motor movements and quality of movement. Consists of 58 items; child is observed in prone, supine, sitting, and standing; takes about 30 min to administer; psychometrics are strong; well researched.
Milani-Comparetti Motor Development Screening Test (Milani-Comparetti and Giodini, 1967)	Birth to 2 years	Criterion-referenced test measuring reflex integration, movement, postural control, and the development of antigravity positions and movement. Quick and easy to administer and score; psychometrics are fair; research is limited.
Infant Neurological Internal Battery (Ellison, 1994)	1–15 months	Norm-referenced, 20-item test measuring neuromotor behavior and competency, including primitive reflexes, hand and head positions, and movement. Quick and easy to administer; normed on 305 infants; reliability and validity measures are fair; research is limited.
Movement Assessment of Infants (Chandler et al., 1980)	2–18 months	Criterion-referenced screening tool, measuring reflexes, muscle tone, automatic reactions, and volitional movement; easy to learn; administration time is approximately 45 min; psychometrics are weak, with few studies of validity and reliability.
Miller Assessment for Preschoolers (Miller, 1988)	2 years, 9 months to 5 years, 8 months	Norm-referenced test measuring foundational sensory and motor abilities, tactile processing kinesthesia, balance, coordination, and motor planning functions; includes some cognitive and language items; has strong psychometric properties; training is recommended; although originally designed as a screening tool, further research supports its use as an evaluation tool.

(Continued)

159

TABLE 4-3 STANDARDIZED TESTS OF SENSORY MOTOR FUNCTIONS, INCLUDING GROSS AND FINE MOTOR SKILLS, POSTURAL CONTROL, SENSORY PROCESSING, AND SENSORY INTEGRATION (*Continued*)

Test Name (Author[s])	Age Range	Purpose/Domains/Description and General Comments
Toddler and Infant Motor Evaluation (Miller and Roid, 1994)	4 months to 3.5 years	Norm-referenced test with eight subtests measuring mobility, stability, motor organization, functional performance, social/emotional abilities, movement component analysis, movement quality, and atypical positions. Complex to administer, but thorough test of quality of movement and postural control; psychometrics are strong.
DeGangi-Berk Test of Sensory Integration (Berk and DeGangi, 1983)	3–5 years	Norm-referenced test consisting of 36 items measuring postural control, bilateral motor co-ordination, and reflex integration. Easy to learn; takes about 30 min to administer; psychometrics are adequate; research is limited.
Sensory Integration and Praxis Tests (Ayres, 1989)	4 years to 8 years, 11 months	Norm-referenced test consisting of 17 tests measuring nonmotor visual perception, various types of praxis, somatosensory processing, vestibular processing, and sensory motor skills. Psychometrics are strong except for test-retest reliability of four tests; extensive training is required; well researched; computer scored.
Sensory Profile (Dunn, 1999); also has infant/toddler and adolescent/adult versions (Brown & Dunn, 2002)	3–12 years	Questionnaire requiring caregivers to rate child behaviors believed to measure aspects of sensory processing, modulation, and emotional/behavioral responses to sensory input. Psychometrics are strong; easy to administer and score.
Test of Sensory Function in Infants (DeGangi and Greenspan, 1989)	4–18 months	Provides an overall measure of sensory processing and reactivity; includes 24 items measuring reactivity to tactile deep pressure and vestibular input, adaptive motor functions, visual-tactile integration, and ocular-motor control. Reliability and validity are adequate.
Touch Inventory for Elementary School-Aged Children (Brasic-Royeen and Fortune, 1990)	Elementary school–aged children	Rating scale for measuring tactile defensiveness. Quick and easy to administer; psycho-metrics are adequate, although research is limited.

Evaluation of Sensory Processing (Parham and Ecker, cited by Bundy, 2002)	Children of all ages	Questionnaire completed by caregivers who are required to rate their child's behaviors on various behaviors believed to measure sensory processing in the following areas: visual, gustatory/olfactory; proprioception, tactile, and vestibular processing. Quick and easy to administer; preliminary research on psychometrics is positive; research is limited.
Quick Neurological Screening Test (Mutti et al., 1978)	5 years through adulthood	Screening tool consisting of 15 test items measuring neurologic functions, including fine and gross motor control, motor planning, spatial organization, visual and auditory perception, and balance. Quick and easy to learn and administer; studies reported in the manual demonstrate adequate reliability and validity.
Peabody Developmental Motor Scales–2 (Folio and Fewell, 2000)	1 month through 6 years	Norm-referenced and criterion-referenced test measuring fine and gross motor skills. Takes about 60 min to administer and is easy to learn; psychometrics are adequate with strong norma-tive data; new version not well researched to date (see review in this chapter).
Bruininks-Oseretsky Test of Motor Proficiency (Bruininks, 1978)	4.5–14.5 years	Norm-referenced test including nine subtests measuring fine and gross motor skills. Validity is strong; reliability measures for composite scores are strong; well researched; takes about 45 min to administer; fairly easy to learn.
Gross Motor Function Measure–Revised (Russell et al., 1993)	5 months to 16 years	Criterion-referenced observational tool designed to measure gross motor functions in children with cerebral palsy and Down's syndrome. Consists of 88 items; administration time is 30–45 min; easy to learn; psychometrics are strong.
Test of Gross Motor Development (Ulrich, 2000)	3–11 years	Norm-referenced assessment measuring basic gross motor skills; includes two subtests: loco-motor and object control. Quick (about 20 min) and easy to administer; psychometrics are ade-quate; not well researched.
Quality of Upper Extremity Skills (Dematteo et al., 1993)	18 months to 8 years	A criterion-referenced tool for evaluating quality of upper extremity movement and hand function in children with cerebral palsy, including dissociated movements, grasp, protective exten-sion, and weight bearing. Easy to administer; psychometrics are strong.

TABLE 4-4 STANDARDIZED ASSESSMENTS OF VISUAL-MOTOR AND VISUAL PERCEPTUAL SKILLS AND HANDWRITING

Test Name (Author[s])	Population	Description/Domains/General Comments	
Development Test of Visual Perception (Hammill et al., 1998)	4–10 years	Norm-referenced tool with eight subtests, including Eye-Hand Coordination, Copying, Spatial Relations, Position in Space, Figure-Ground, Visual Closure, Visual-Motor Speed, and Form Constancy. Administration time is about 30–40 min; measures both visual perception and visual-motor integration skills in children; strong normative data, reliability, and validity.	
Beery-Buktenica Developmental Test of Visual-Motor Integration (Beery, 1997)	3–18 years of age	Norm-referenced design copy test. Quick and easy to administer; this edition includes a nonmotor visual perceptual screening and a motor coordination screening test; psychometric properties are strong.	
Test of Visual-Motor Skills–Revised (Gardner, 1995)	3–14 years of age	Norm-referenced design copy test. Quick and easy to administer. Unique in that type of errors are classified and scored to give qualitative information; psychometric properties are adequate; quick and easy to administer.	
Test of Visual-Perceptual Skills (Gardner, 1997) (has a similar test for children 12–18 years)	4–13 years of age	Norm-referenced test of visual perception measuring figure ground, spatial relations, visual memory and visual sequential memory, visual form constancy, visual closure, and visual discrimination. Quick and easy to administer; psychometrics are adequate.	

Motor-Free Visual Perception Test–Revised (Colarussi and Hammill, 1995)	4–12 years of age	Norm-referenced test of visual perception measuring figure ground, spatial relations, visual memory and visual closure, and visual discrimination. Quick and easy to administer; psychometrics are adequate.
Evaluation Tool of Children's Handwriting (Amundson, 1995)	Grades 1–6	Criterion-referenced tool measuring cursive and manuscript handwriting, including alphabet and number writing, copying, dictation, and sentence generation. It assesses legibility, pencil grasp and pressure, hand preference, manipulative skills with the writing tool, and classroom performance; easy to learn; psychometrics are adequate.
Minnesota Handwriting Assessment (Reisman, 1999)	First- and second-grade students	Criterion-referenced test measuring cursive and manuscript handwriting, including speed, legibility, form, alignment with baseline, size, and letter and word space. Research is limited, although research to date supports reliability and validity; easy to administer.

TABLE 4-5 ASSESSMENT TOOLS FOR EVALUATING PSYCHOLOGICAL, PSYCHOSOCIAL, AND EMOTIONAL AREAS IN CHILDREN[a]

Test Name (Author[s])	Age Range	Description and Purpose
Early Coping Inventory (Zeitlin et al., 1988)	Infants and toddlers	Observational instrument that evaluates sensorimotor organization, reactive behaviors, and self-initiated behaviors, all believed to be important for effective coping.
Neonatal Behavioral Assessment Scale (Brazelton, 1984)	Infants	Rating scale that assesses reflex behavior and motor maturity, responses to sensory stimuli, temperament, and adapting and coping strategies.
Functional Emotional Assessment Scale (Greenspan et al., 1996)	3–48 months	Evaluates emotional and social capacities throughout different stages of sensory motor and cognitive development; a rating scale to assist in organizing and interpreting unstructured observations of the child and the child with his or her caregiver(s).
Temperament and Atypical Behavior Scales (Bagnato et al., 1999)	Birth to 3 years of age	Rating scale measuring sensory regulation and attachment behaviors.
KidCOTE (cited by Kunz and Brayman, 1999)	Children and adolescents with psychiatric illness	Performance-based instrument evaluating behaviors in four areas: general behaviors, sensory motor performance, cognitive behaviors, and psychosocial behaviors.

Vineland Adaptive Behavior Scales (Sparrow et al., 1984)	Birth through 18 years of age	Measures communication, daily living skills, socialization, and motor skills. Uses a behavior rating scale that is completed through a structured parent interview.
Adolescent Role Assessment (Black, 1976)	Adolescents	Structured interview and rating scale that evaluates childhood play, socialization within the family, school functioning, socialization with peers, occupational choice, and anticipated adult work.
Gardner Social Development Scale (Gardner and Gardner, 1994)	Children	Parent questionnaire; norm-referenced assessment of social skills.
Social Adjustment Inventory for Children and Adolescents (John et al.,1987)	Children and adolescents	Semistructured parent interview examining patterns of social function in school, community, and home environments.
Social Skills Rating System (Gresham and Elliot, 1990)	Preschool; grades K–7; grades 7–12	Standardized norm-referenced scales including parent, teacher, and child forms; examines social behavior and relationships.

[a]Not all of the assessment tools listed in this table are standardized.

TABLE 4-6	ASSESSMENT TOOLS FOR EVALUATING CONTEXTUAL ELEMENTS

Title (Author[s])	Description and Purpose
Assessment of Home Environments (Yarrow et al., 1975)	Designed to be used for early intervention; structured observations; examines qualities of the home environment of infants for promoting development.
Child Care Centre Accessibility Checklist (Metro Toronto Community Services, 1991)	Examines and measures the level of barrier-free accessibility of child care environments.
Classroom Environment Index (Stern and Walker, 1971)	A self-administered questionnaire examining the student's perception of the classroom environment and the student-environment fit.
Classroom Observation Guide (Griswold, 1994)	An observational guide that examines qualities of activities, people, and communication patterns in a classroom environment.
Environment Assessment Index (Poresky, 1987)	Questionnaire format completed by structured observations and interview; examines characteristics of home environments for children aged 3–11 years living in rural areas for promoting education and development.
Home Observation for the Measurement of the Environment–Revised (Caldwell and Bradley, 1984)	Structured observations and interview format; examines physical, social, and cultural contexts of the home environment of children from birth to 6 years of age.
Infant/Toddler Environment Rating Scale (Harms et al, 1990)	Examines the quality of child care environments for children up to 30 months; based on structured observations.
Person-Environment Fit Scale (Coulton, 1979)	Self-report questionnaire measuring person-environmental fit through the examination of physical, social, and cultural contexts.

sensory integration functions; (4) assessments measuring visual-motor and visual perceptual skills and handwriting; (5) assessments measuring psychosocial functioning; and (6) contextual assessments, including ecologic inventories.

EXAMINER RESPONSIBILITIES AND ETHICAL CONSIDERATIONS

Your responsibilities as an examiner or standardized test administrator cannot be underestimated because critical decisions such as eligibility for certain programs are sometimes made based on your test results. Responsibilities include issues surrounding **competency** and **ethics**. Competency in the administration of standardized tests to children requires an understanding of child development (see Chapter 3), knowledge of the principles of measurement, and the ability to effectively interact and establish rapport with children of various ages and personalities.

Learning to administer a standardized test is a labor-intensive process. Developing competency involves first reading and thoroughly understanding the content in the test manual. It is important to understand the test development processes, its purposes, the strengths and characteristics of the normative data, reliability and validity, and the technical aspects of test administration and scoring. Examples of therapists administering standardized tests to children are depicted in Figures 4-1, 4-2, and 4-3. Some standardized tests require a certification process or require therapists to go through a formal training program. However, many can be self-taught provided that you have the background knowledge in child development and measurement and are willing to put the time in to read the manual carefully, learn the administration and scoring procedures, and then practice. Observing experienced therapists administer tests is another learning strategy that is often helpful.

Competency guidelines or **standards of practice** related to the use of standardized assessments are provided by professional organizations such as the American Occupational Therapy Association (AOTA) and by legislation such as the Individuals With Disabilities Education Act (1997) (see Table 4-7). Organizations that sell testing materials, such as Western Psychological Services and the Psychological Corporation, also have competency standards and qualification forms that potential users must complete to purchase certain materials. These standards are consistent with the Standards for Educational and Psy-

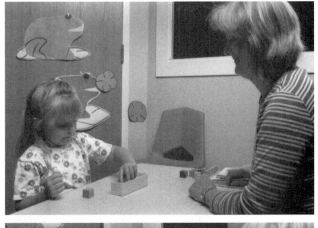

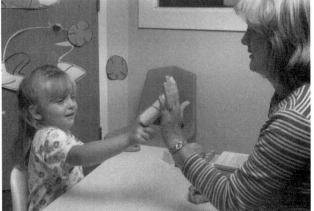

Figure 4-1 Therapist administering a standardized test to a child.

chological Testing published the American Psychological Association and prepared by the American Psychological Association in collaboration with the American Educational Research Association and the National Council on Measurement in Education.

You also must abide by the **AOTA's Code of Ethics** (AOTA, 1994a) throughout all aspects of your services, and some specific content applies to the use of standardized testing (see Appendix E, 1-2, 1-3, 4-1, 4-4, and 5-1). It is important for you to understand the purposes and limitations of the tests that you use. For test scores to be valid, tests must be administered in the standardized

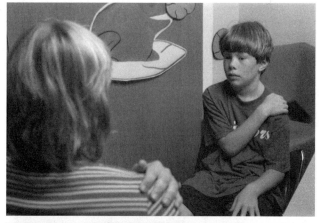

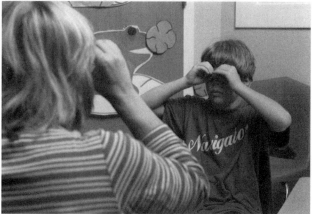

Figure 4-2 Therapist administering a standardized test to a child.

manner detailed in the manual. If you must deviate from the standardized procedures to accommodate for child needs or limitations, you must disclose this in your evaluation report and interpret scores cautiously. You may decide to use descriptive interpretations only instead of reporting the scores. Assessment information obtained through administration of the test can still be valuable as clinical observation data and can be used in the interpretation process. It is also important (as always) to respect client rights, including matters related to confidentiality and the client's right of refusal to participate in or agree to procedures.

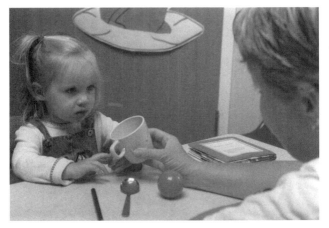

Figure 4-3 Therapist administering a standardized test to a child.

INTERPRETATION OF STANDARD SCORES FROM NORM-REFERENCED ASSESSMENTS

The first step in scoring a child's performance on a test is to obtain a **raw score**. The raw score is then converted to a **standard score** so that meaningful interpretations can be made. A standard score takes into consideration how your client did in relation to the scores of children in the normative sample with whom he or she is compared. The scores of children in the **normative sample** typically follow a normal distribution, with the bulk of scores clustered around the mean and relatively few scores falling at the extreme ends of the range. The test manual will include tables (often they are in the back of the test manual) to convert your raw scores to standard scores.

The **standard deviation** (SD) of a population is a measure of variability or the spread of scores (the extent to which scores deviate from the mean and from one another), and SD is used to divide up the normal distribution (see Fig. 4-4). In a normal distribution, approximately 68% of the scores are within 1 SD of the mean, 28% between 1 and 2 SD of the mean, and 4% outside 2 SD of the mean. This is important because it is believed that "typical" or "normal" performance is behavior (or test scores) that fall within 1 to 1.5 SDs from the mean. In

TABLE 4-7	PROFESSIONAL STANDARDS RELATED TO STANDARDIZED TESTING

Source	Standards
American Occupational Therapy Association, 1998	Standard IV: Assessment 4. Occupational therapy assessment methods shall be appropriate to the individual's age and developmental level; gender; education; socioeconomic and ethnic background; medical status; and functional abilities.... 5. An occupational therapy practitioner shall follow accepted protocols when standardized tests are used. Standardized tests are tests whose scores are based on accompanying normative data that may reflect age ranges, gender, ethnic groups, geographic regions, and SES status. If standardized tests are not available or appropriate, the results shall be expressed in descriptive reports, and standardized scales shall not be used.
Individuals With Disabilities Education Act, 1997	In conducting the evaluation, the local educational agency shall use a variety of assessment tools and strategies to gather relevant functional and developmental information...; use technically sound instruments that may assess the relative contribution of cognitive and behavioral factors, in addition to physical or developmental factors. Each local educational agency shall ensure that tests and other evaluation materials used to assess a child are selected and administered so as not to be discriminatory on a racial or cultural basis; and are provided and administered in the child's native language or other mode of communication, unless it is clearly not feasible to do so; and any standardized tests that are given to the child have been validated for the specific purpose for which they are used; are administered by trained and knowledgeable personnel; and are administered in accordance with any instructions provided by the producer of such tests.

SES, socioeconomic status.

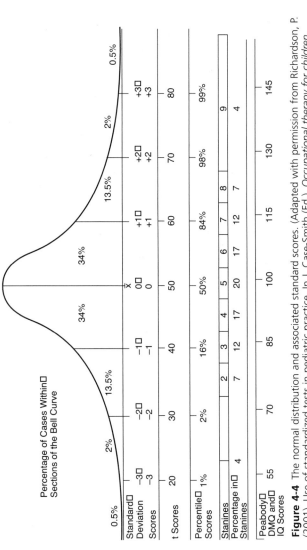

Figure 4-4 The normal distribution and associated standard scores. (Adapted with permission from Richardson, P. (2001). Use of standardized tests in pediatric practice. In J. Case-Smith (Ed.), *Occupational therapy for children.* (4th ed.). St. Louis, MO: Mosby, 2001:226.)

other words, if you consider a score 1 SD below the mean to be significantly below average, you believe that when a child performs at or below the performance of 16% of the children in the comparative normative group then the child's performance is considered to be lower than the range of scores considered to be typical or average.

Common standard scores used to report a child's results on pediatric assessment tools are *z* **scores** (mean = 0, SD = 1), *t* **scores** (mean = 50, SD = 10), and standard scores such as IQ scores (mean = 100, SD =15). **Stanine scores**, which range from 1 to 9 (with a mean of 5 and scores of 3–7 interpreted as being within the "normal" range) are also sometimes used. As long as you know the mean and SD of the sample that is used to compare your score, you can convert from one type of standard score to another (see the examples in Box 4-2) because they are all based on a normal distribution.

Percentile scores are defined as the percentage of people in the standardization sample or population who scored at or below a given score. For example, if your child's raw score of 15 was converted to a percentile score of 38, that means that 38% of the children that he or she is compared with scored at or below your child's score. As

---

BOX 4-2	CONVERTING STANDARD SCORES TO *Z* SCORES

Example 1. Standard score = 7, from a test with a mean of 15, and standard deviation = 5

$$z \text{ score} = \frac{\text{observed standard score} - \text{mean}}{\text{standard deviation}}$$

$$= \frac{7 - 15}{5}$$

z score = −1.6, significantly below average performance

Example 2. Given a *t* score of 65 (mean = 50, standard deviation = 10)

$$z \text{ score} = \frac{\text{observed standard score} - \text{mean}}{\text{standard deviation}}$$

$$= \frac{65 - 50}{10}$$

z score = 1.5, significantly above average performance

with other standard scores, percentile scores are derived based on the normal distribution. The mean, therefore, is at the fiftieth percentile, and percentile scores within 1 SD of the mean are those that range from the sixteenth percentile to the eighty-fourth percentile (Fig. 4-4).

Another type of score sometimes reported is an **age-equivalent score**. An age-equivalent score relates the child's score to that of a typical or average child of a particular age group. For example, if a child's raw score of 25 is converted to an age-equivalent score of 6 years, 4 months, this means that the child received the mean score for children aged 6 years, 4 months (from the normative sample) or is performing like typical children aged 6 years, 4 months. Methods of reporting the results of standardized assessments, including test scores, are provided in the sample evaluation reports included in Chapter 7.

STANDARD ERROR OF MEASUREMENT

All test scores are really made up of three components: the **observed score** (the score the child obtained), the **true score** (the hypothetical construct, representing what the child's score would be if it reflected the child's true ability), and **measurement error**. The child's observed score is the sum of the measurement error plus the true score (Carmines and Zeller, 1979). Measurement error is inevitable with standardized testing and can result from characteristics of the test itself, examiner error, and child errors (see Table 4-8).

Standard error of measurement (SEM) indicates how much variability can be attributed to error (Murphy and Davidshofer, 1988) and depends on (1) the test-retest reliability coefficient, "r" (discussed later in this chapter), and (2) the SD of the sample used to determine the reliability coefficient. It is calculated using the following formula: $\text{SEM} = \text{SD}\sqrt{1 - \text{r}}$.

The SEM is important in relation to test scores because sometimes test scores are reported using the SEM to account for the test's measurement error. A test's SEM usually is reported in the test manual, and it can be used to create a confidence interval around a child's observed

TABLE 4-8	TYPES OF MEASUREMENT ERROR

Error Type	Description
Child errors	Lack of understanding of directions; noncompliance; inability to give "typical" or "true" performance owing to fatigue, disinterest, illness, or inattention; lack of motivation; may also "overachieve" owing to ability to perform better in a one-on-one situation, eager to please administrator; practice effect if test is given more than once.
	Test-retest reliability coefficients are one measure of the degree of possible child errors.
Examiner errors	Inability to put the child at ease or to establish rapport with the child; poor optimization of the testing environment; lack of competency, resulting in inaccurate test administration procedures, including presentation of verbal directions and test items, use of materials and testing protocols; scoring errors
	Interrater reliability coefficients are one measure of the degree of possible examiner errors.
Test characteristic errors	Damaged testing materials, poorly calibrated testing materials, or use of substitute, nonstandardized materials; lack of objectivity or clarity of scoring criteria; high complexity of test administration procedures.
	Reflected to some degree by both interrater and test-retest reliability coefficients.

score. A confidence interval is a range in which it can be stated with a known degree of confidence that a specific score would fall. Based on the normal distribution, it is known that 68% of scores fall within 1 SD of the mean and that 95% of scores fall between -2.5 and $+2.5$ SD of the mean. Therefore, we can use these numbers to construct 68% and 95% confidence intervals.

For example, suppose a child 6 years of age had an observed standard score on the Beery-Buktenica Developmental Test of Visual-Motor Integration (Beery, 1997) of 70 (mean = 100, SD = 15) and the manual reports that the SEM for this test is 6 for a child of that age. Instead of reporting the child's score as 70, it is more precise to express the score in terms of a confidence interval by stating that you are 68% confident that the child's true score falls between 64 and 76. To establish the 95% confidence interval, you add and subtract 2 SEMs instead of 1 and report the child's true score as falling within the range of 58 to 82.

EVALUATING PSYCHOMETRIC PROPERTIES OF ASSESSMENT TOOLS

Evaluating the **psychometric properties** of standardized assessment tools involves reading carefully and critiquing evidence in the test manual and from other studies published in referred journals related to normative data, reliability, and validity. Before addressing how to evaluate a test's normative data, reliability, and validity, a type of statistic—the correlation coefficient—is briefly discussed because this statistic is frequently used by test developers to establish reliability and validity.

A **correlation coefficient** is a measure of the strength of the relationship between two variables. It is a number that ranges from −1 (a perfect negative relationship) to +1 (a perfect positive correlation), and a correlation of zero means that there is no relationship. A negative correlation means that as one variable increases, the other decreases (or vice versa). A positive correlation means that as one variable increases, the other increases, or as one decreases, the other decreases. In other words, if both variables move in the same direction, it is a positive correlation, and if they move in opposite directions, the correlation or relationship is negative. Examples of correlations are given in Table 4-9. In general, weak correlation coefficients range from 0.26 to 0.49 (or −0.26 to −0.49), moderate correlation coefficients from 0.50 to 0.69 (or −0.50 to −0.69), and strong correlations from 0.7 to 1 (or from −0.7 to −1) (Munro, 2001). However, few hard and fast "rules" about determining the clinical significance of the correlation have been developed (although you can conduct a

TABLE 4-9 | EXAMPLES OF CORRELATION COEFFICIENTS

Variables	Correlation Coefficient	Interpretation
Changes in ratings of hand function were correlated with changes in performance on the COPM after occupational therapy treatment	r = 0.28 (Law et al., 1994)	Weak, positive relationship suggesting that changes on the COPM are not strongly related to changes in hand function
Scores of 10-year-old children on the TVMS (Gardner, 1995) were correlated with scores of 10-year-old children on the Beery-Buktenica Developmental Test of VMI (Beery, 1997)	r = 0.56 (Gardner, 1995)	Moderate positive correlation, suggesting that children score similarly on these two tests; as scores increase on the TVMS, they also increase on the VMI; as they decrease on the TVMS, they tend to decrease on the VMI
On the Klein-Bell ADL Scale (Klein and Bell, 1982), predictive validity indicated a relationship between hospital discharge scores and number of hours of daily assistance required at home	r = −0.86	Strong negative correlation, indicating that as scores on the Klein-Bell increased (indicating higher levels of ADL function), the number of hours of daily assistance from others decreased
Test-retest reliability coefficient of the Constructional Praxis of the SIPT (children were tested twice within 1–2 weeks, and their scores were correlated)	r = 0.70 (Ayres, 1989)	Moderate to strong positive correlation, indicating that children's score similarly when tested twice; as a measure of test-retest reliability, this correlation is fair.

ADLs, activities of daily living; COPM, Canadian Occupational Performance Measure; SIPT, Sensory Integration and Praxis Tests; TVMS, Test of Visual-Motor Skills; VMI, Visual-Motor Integration.

test to determine statistical significance). Therefore, determining acceptable correlation values when evaluating research studies that examine the reliability and validity of standardized tests is somewhat subjective. A format for completing reviews of standardized tests is provided in Figure 4-5. Two sample reviews of frequently used standardized assessment tools, including reviews of the Pedi-

---

Standardized Assessment Review Form

Name of Test:
Author(s) and Publisher:
Cost:

Test Description:
(Purpose[s]; Age Range; Domains Evaluated; Type and Format; Summarize Test Development Process; Administration Time)

Psychometric Properties:
    Reliability:

  ❑ Validity:

    Normative Date:

Practical Considerations:
(Technical Skill/Training Required; Time, Space, and Materials Required; Client Prerequisite Skills)

Overall Strengths and Weaknesses:

Reference List (list other sources of data about the test published in refereed journals):

Figure 4-5 Sample review form for evaluating standardized assessment tools.

atric Evaluation of Disability Inventory (Haley et al., 1992), and the Peabody Developmental Motor Scales–2 (Folio and Fewell, 2000), are provided at the end of this chapter.

Evaluation of the Normative Data

Norms provided in a test manual are not the "true norms" but rather estimates of the true norms based on the performance of the sample population used to develop the norms. Therefore, the usefulness of normative data is directly related to how much the sample used to generate the norms reflects its intended population. This is also true for criterion-referenced tests. Typically, criteria are developed based on the performance of a sample from the population of interest. Therefore, the sample used must be considered, particularly in relation to age, gender, disability, and sociocultural factors, when determining how relevant the test items and criteria are for your clients.

When evaluating how good normative data are, the first question you need to ask is, "How representative is the sample used to generate the normative data of the population that the test was designed for?" For example, if a test was designed to target U.S. children, then the sample should be selected using a stratified, randomized procedure to ensure that age, race, gender, socioeconomic status, and urban and rural populations are all represented, and in approximately the same proportions as in the U.S. population. It is also important that the sample you are using to compare your client's performance is relevant for your purposes. A relevant sample is one that has characteristics similar to the clients with whom you intend to use the test. Norms should also be relatively recent. It is important that you take the time to review the methods used to obtain the sample, which should be covered in detail in the test manual. Generally, the more recent the norms the better (ideally within 10 years) and the larger the normative sample the better; samples obtained through a randomized process are more representative of populations being targeted than convenient samples.

Reliability

A reliable assessment tool is one that is consistent, i.e., designed in such a way that all those who administer the test to the same individual under the same set of circumstances would obtain the same results. In addition, if the test is reliable, then children who are asked to do the test items should perform in a relatively consistent manner if given the test more than once within a reasonably short period (days or a couple of weeks). The SEM discussed earlier is one measure of **reliability**. There are three other types of reliability that you should look for when evaluating the overall reliability of an assessment tool: interrater, test-retest, and internal consistency. To evaluate how reliable an assessment tool is, review research studies reported in the test manual designed to evaluate all three of these types of reliability. Similar studies may also have been published in refereed journals after the test was published and are also important sources of information about a test's reliability.

Interrater Reliability

Interrater reliability, also referred to as interrater agreement, examines the extent to which test results vary because of factors introduced into the testing situation by the test administrators. Typically, interrater reliability studies determine the correlation between the scores of two independent raters scoring the same child simultaneously. Interrater reliability is especially important when scoring involves some degree of subjectivity. If a test has strong interrater reliability, then two different raters (with adequate training in the test administration and scoring procedures) scoring the same child should get exactly the same results. There is no universal agreement as to how high the minimum acceptable interrater reliability coefficient should be, and factors such as the type of behaviors being measured and the range of possible scores should be taken into consideration. A standard was suggested by Anastasi (1988) of 0.80; however, specifically for the types of tests we use in pediatric occupational therapy, minimum values of acceptability for interrater reliability tend to be closer to 0.90.

Test-Retest Reliability

Test-retest reliability refers to how consistently a group a children will perform on the same test when it is given on more than one occasion (usually just twice) in a relatively short period. Scores from the two testing situations are correlated with one another and represent a measure of stability of the test results over the time interval. Essentially, a test with good test-retest reliability assures you that if you gave a test to a child and then gave it to the child again (within a couple of days or weeks) he or she would perform similarly, generating similar scores. When evaluating an assessment tool's research related to test-retest reliability, look for the number of subjects used in the study (should be >20, and the more the better) and the length of time between testing (should be 1–2 weeks). Test-retest correlation coefficients tend to be stronger when there is a shorter interval between testing. Again, there are no hard and fast, definitive rules about what the minimal acceptable correlation coefficients should be. It is important to note that the stability of the behaviors being measured greatly impacts the test-retest reliability. For example, fine motor skills would not be expected to vary naturally near as much as social behavior, mood, or ability to attend. It is important in pediatric assessments that the interval is not too long because developmental changes could naturally occur, or too short, which would allow the children to remember the items, potentially causing a practice effect. A practice effect occurs when children tend to score slightly higher the second time because of their previous experience. In general, acceptable coefficients for test-retest reliability are those greater than 0.8 (King-Thomas and Hacker, 1987).

Internal Consistency

A test is believed to have **internal consistency** when the individual test items correlate with one another to a certain degree. For example, if a test is designed to measure fine motor ability, then, in theory, all of the test items should be related to or be able to measure some aspect of fine motor performance. Therefore, a child (whether he or she has strong or weak fine motor skills) should perform somewhat similarly on all of the test items that measure this area. Studies of internal consistency often will correlate a group of scores from one half of the test with those from the other half (first half with second half; odd- versus even-numbered items), also referred to as split-half reliability.

Various more sophisticated statistical techniques are commonly used to calculate reliability coefficients for measuring internal consistency (e.g., Kuder-Richardson and Cronbach's alpha) (Green, 1991) that specifically account for the ways of grouping the test items and for allowing the total length of the test to be considered in the analysis (i.e., the split-half method reduces the test length in half, which would result in a slightly lower coefficient than if the whole test was accounted for in the calculation). High correlations indicate that the test is measuring a homogeneous construct. If the test has good internal consistency, then correlation coefficients should be between 0.6 and 0.8 (Anastasi, 1988).

Validity

Validity may simply be referred to as the extent to which a test actually measures what it was intended to measure. However, it is really a much more complex idea than it seems. For example, on what type of evidence may we interpret test scores to be a good indication of social function? Of gross motor skill? Of sensory processing? How well does a kindergarten readiness test predict success or failure in early elementary school? Can we justifiably allow or disallow a child to enroll in a specific program based on his or her test scores? What evidence is there to support the interpretations of the test scores that we make and how we use them?

Messick (1995) defined validity as an integrated, evaluative judgment of the degree to which empirical evidence and theoretical rationales support the adequacy and appropriateness of our inferences and actions based on test scores or other modes of assessment. He further emphasized the importance of the meaning, relevance, clinical utility, and value implications of scores as a basis for action and the functional worth of scores in terms of the social consequences of their use. Test validation, then, is scientific inquiry into score meaning. Although Messick emphasized that validity is a unitary idea, different types of validity (content, criterion related, and construct) have been described in the literature, and these different types are often addressed separately in test manuals of pediatric standardized assessments. Therefore, each of these facets of validity is discussed separately in the following subsections; however, it is important to note that they overlap greatly and that they all contribute evidence addressing the issue of score meaning.

Content Validity

Content validity is the extent to which the test items of a particular test adequately and accurately sample the skill areas or behaviors it is designed to measure while not being contaminated by items measuring other types of behaviors or skills. For example, if a test is designed to measure fine motor performance, there should be enough items for adequately measuring all aspects of fine motor skill (such as eye-hand coordination, speed and dexterity, grasp patterns, visual motor control, and functional fine motor tasks). There should be evidence in the manual that items addressing all facets of fine motor skill were systematically analyzed and then the best items were selected. It is never feasible to include all possible test items, which would make tests too long. Often, evidence for selecting adequate test content is derived from a panel of experts who determine how each test item relates to each domain being tested and comment on the thoroughness of the items for measuring each of the domains/constructs the test is designed to measure. Then, statistical techniques are used to analyze the items and to help select the "best" or most meaningful items. A table of specifications may be included in the test manual to summarize how test items relate to each of the domains, and there should be a description in the manual regarding the selection process, with a clear rationale for the test items that were ultimately selected.

Construct Validity

Construct validity addresses the extent to which the test measures the construct or domain being measured. Common constructs measured in pediatric occupational therapy include fine motor performance, gross motor function, sensory integration, sensory processing, play, self-help skills, self-esteem, social skills, and visual perception. These constructs, for the most part (and some more than others), are abstract entities that cannot be measured directly. For example, a test of sensory processing really measures directly behaviors that are theoretically believed to represent sensory processing, since we cannot measure this brain function directly. When a test is developed, hypotheses are generated about the relationship among variables believed to be measured by the test. Several sources of evidence are necessary to evaluate construct validity, which examines the theory supporting the domains being tested.

One source of evidence comes from studies comparing the performance of a sample of children on the test with their scores on a similar test. For example, the Test of Visual Motor Skills–Revised (Gardner, 1995) and the Beery-Buktenica Developmental Test of Visual-Motor Integration (Beery, 1997) both state that they measure visual-motor skills. Therefore, children should perform similarly (their scores should correlate positively) on these tests (see Table 4-3).

Another source of evidence of construct validity comes from studies that compare scores from different groups of children. For example, on tests measuring areas of development, it would be expected that the scores of older children would reflect a higher level of performance than the scores of younger children. Similarly, the scores from typical children would be expected to be higher than those from children with known developmental delays.

Research applying multivariate statistical techniques, particularly grouping techniques such as factor and cluster analyses, also provide evidence for construct validity. Examples of standardized tests that have been studied extensively using these techniques include the Sensory Integration and Praxis Tests (Ayres, 1989, Mulligan 1998, 2000) and the Sensory Profile (Dunn, 1999). The purpose of factor analysis is to group tests that are alike or that all relate to some underlying construct, whereas cluster analysis groups scores of children who score similarly.

Criterion-Related Validity

Criterion-related validity is the ability of a test to predict performance on other measures or activities. A test may have predictive validity (ability to predict future performance on some criterion) or concurrent validity (the ability to predict present performance on some criterion). To evaluate concurrent validity, the scores of a sample of children are correlated with performance on the criterion measure. For example, if a test of visual motor skills is believed to predict handwriting performance, then scores on the visual motor test would be expected to be positively correlated with scores on a test that measures handwriting ability.

Predictive validity studies examine the relationship between a current test score and performance on some criterion measured in the future. For example, it is of interest to occupational therapists and other child development experts to identify infants and preschool children who are at risk for developmental problems or for school problems once they reach school age. Through early identification (using a test of development that can predict reasonably well whether a child is at risk for developing problems later in life), early intervention services can be provided.

IMPORTANT CONSIDERATIONS AND CHALLENGES RELATED TO THE USE OF STANDARDIZED TESTS

The development and use of standardized tests in pediatric occupational therapy is quite extensive and has allowed for a more scientific, objective approach to evaluation. Although the use of standardized tests enhances the credibility of our profession, these tests are not without drawbacks. First, many tests are expensive, and it may be labor intensive to become competent in their use. Second, young children are often difficult to test due to behavioral problems such as inattention, inability to comprehend directions, or noncompliance. Third, many tests were normed on typical children instead of on the clinical populations often seen by occupational therapists, which limits their use, particularly for evaluating client progress. Fourth, some standardized tests are limited in their usefulness for developing intervention programs, and, for some populations, such as children with severe and profound disabilities, relatively few tests are available. Fifth, when reporting scores, it is important to be able to explain standardized test scores in language that can be easily understood by all interested parties, such as parents and teachers.

SUMMARY

This chapter provided information about the use of standardized assessment tools, including factors to consider when selecting specific tests and how to evaluate the psychometric properties of a test. The interpretation of standardized test scores was covered in detail. Ethical and professional considerations were discussed, and lists of available pediatric standardized assessment tools organized by skill area were provided.

Although standardized assessment tools provide useful, objective assessment information, test scores should never be a substitute for sound clinical judgment and should be viewed as just one source of data to be used as you engage in the interpretation process of your evaluation.

References

American Occupational Therapy Association (1998). Standards of practice for occupational therapy. *American Journal of Occupational Therapy, 52*, 866–869.

American Occupational Therapy Association (1994). Occupational therapy code of ethics. *American Journal of Occupational Therapy, 48*, 1037–1038.

Amundson, S. J. (1995). *Evaluation tool of children's handwriting (ETCH)*. Homer, AK: O.T. Kids Inc.

Anastasi, A. (1988). *Psychological testing* (5th ed.). New York, NY: Macmillan.

Ayres, A. J. (1989). *Sensory integration and praxis tests*. Los Angeles, CA: Western Psychological Services.

Bagnato, S., Neisworth, J. T., Salvia, J. Hunt, J. (1999). *Temperament and atypical behavior scales*. Baltimore, MD: Brookes Publisher.

Baron & Curtin (1999). Reliability of the self-assessment of occupational functioning. *American Journal of Occupational Therapy, 53*(5), 482–488.

Bates-Ames, L., Gillespie, C., Haines, A. B., & Ilg, F. (1980). *Gesell preschool test*. Rosemont, NJ: Gesell Institute of Human Development, Programs for Education, Inc.

Bayley, N. (1993). *Bayley scales of infant development* (2nd ed.). San Antonio, TX: The Psychological Corp.

Beery, K. (1997). *Beery-Buktenica developmental test of visual-motor integration (VMI)* (4th ed.). Parsippany, NJ: Modern Curriculun Press.

Berk R., DeGangi, G. (1983). DeGangi-Berk Test of Sensory Integration. Los Angeles: Western Psychological Services.

Black, M. (1976). Adolescent role assessment. *American Journal of Occupational Therapy 30*, 73–79.

Brasic-Royeen, C. B., & Fortune, J. C. (1990). TIE: Touch inventory for school-aged children. *American Journal of Occupational Therapy, 44*, 155–160.

Brazelton, T. B. (1984). *The neonatal behavioral assessment scale*. Philadelphia, PA: J. B. Lippincott.

Brown, C. & Dunn, W. (2002). *Sensory profile: Adolescent/adult version*. San Antonio, TX: The Psychological Corporation.

Bruininks, R. H. (1978). *Bruininks-Oseretsky test of motor proficiency*. Circle Pines, MN: American Guidance Service.

Bundy, A. (2002). Clinical observation of neuromotor performance, evaluation of sensory processing and touch inventory for elementary school children. In A. Bundy, S., Lane, E. Murray (Eds.), *Sensory integration theory and practice* (2nd ed., pp. 191–198). Philadelphia, PA: F.A. Davis Company.

Bundy, A. (1997). Play and playfulness: What to look for. In L. D. Parham & L. S. Fazzio (Eds.), *Play in occupational therapy for children* (pp. 52–66). St. Louis, MO: Mosby–Year Book.

Caldwell, B. M., & Bradley, R. H. (1984). *Home observation for the measurement of the environment* (Rev. Ed.). Little Rock, AK: University of Arkansas.

Campbell, S. (1989). Measurement in developmental therapy: Past, present and future. *Physical and Occupational Therapy in Pediatrics, 9*, 1–13.

Carmines, E. G., & Zeller, R. A. (1979). *Reliability and validity assessment*. Newbury Park: Sage.

Chandler, L., Andrews, M., & Swanson, M. (1980). *Movement assessment of infants*. Rolling Bay, WA.

Colarussi, R., & Hammill, D. (1995). *The motor free visual perception test–revised*. Novato, CA: Academic Therapy Publications.

Coster, W., Deeney, T., Haltiwanger, J., & Haley, S. (1998). *School Function Assessment (SFA)*. San Antonio, TX: Psychological Corp.

Coulton, C. J. (1979). Developing an instrument to measure person-environment fit. *Journal of Social Service Research, 3,* 159–173.

DeGangi, G. A., & Greenspan, S. I. (1989). *Test of sensory function in infants.* Los Angeles: Western Psychological Services.

Ellison, P. (1994). *The INFANIB: A reliable method for the neuromotor assessment of infants.* Tucson, AZ: Therapy Skill Builders.

Dematteo, C., Law, M., Russell, D., Pollack, N., Rosenbaum, P., & Walter, S. (1993). The reliability and validity of the quality of upper extremity skills test. *Physical and Occupational Therapy in Pediatrics, 13*(2), 1–18.

Dunn, W. (1999). *Sensory profile, user's manual.* San Antonio, TX: The Psychological Corporation.

Fisher A. G. (1999). *Assessment of motor and process skills* (3rd ed.). Fort Collins, CO: Three Star Press.

Fisher, A. G., & Bryze, K. (1997). *School AMPS: School version of the assessment of motor and process skills.* Ft. Collins, CO: Three Star Press.

Fisher, A. G. (1994). *Assessment of motor and process skills manual* (research edition 7.0) Unpublished test manual. Fort Collins, CO: Colorado State University.

Folio, R. & Fewell, R. (2000). Peabody Developmental Motor Scales-2, (2nd ed.). Austin, TX: Pro-Ed.

Frankenburg, W. K., & Dodds, J. (1992). *Denver II, screening manual.* Denver, CO: Denver Developmental Materials, Inc.

Furuno, S. O'Reilly, K., Hosaka, C.M., Zeisloft, B., & Allman, T. (1984). *The Hawaii Early Learning Profile.* Palo Alto, CA: VORT.

Gardner, M. & Gardner, K. (1994). *Gardner social development scale.* Hydesville, CA: Psychological and Educational Publications Inc.

Gardner, M. (1995). *Test of visual-motor skills–revised.* Hydesville, CA: Psychological and Educational Publications Inc.

Gardner, M. (1997). *Test of visual-perceptual skills (non-motor)–revised.* Hydesville, CA: Psychological and Educational Publications Inc.

Gilfoyle, E. (1981). *Training: Occupational therapy education management in the schools.* Bethesda, MD: AOTA.

Green, K. E. (1991). Reliability, validity, and test score interpretation. In K.E. Green (Ed.), *Educational testing: Issues and applications* (pp. 27–38). New York, NY: Garland.

Greenspan, S., DeGangi, G., & Wieder, S. (1996). *Functional emotional assessment scale.* Bethesda, MD: The Interdisciplinary Council on Developmental and Learning Disorders.

Gresham, F., & Elliot, S. (1990). Social skills rating system. Circle Pines, MN: American Guidance Service Inc.

Griswold, L. (1994). Ethnographic analysis: A study of classroom environments. *American Journal of Occupational Therapy,* 48(5), 397–402.

Haley, S., Coster, W., Ludlow, L., Haltiwanger, J., & Andrellos, P. (1992). *Pediatric evaluation of disability inventory.* San Antonio, TX: Psychological Corp.

Hammill, D., Pearson, N. A., & Voress, J. K. (1998). *Developmental test of visual perception (DVPT-2).* Austin, TX: ProED.

Hamilton, B. B., & Granger, C. U. (1991). *Functional Independence Measure for Children (Wee-FIM).* Buffalo, NY: Research Foundation of the State University of New York.

Individuals with Disabilities Education Act (IDEA) Amendments of 1997 (PL.105-17). U.S.C. 1400.

John, K., Gammon, G. D., Prusoff, B. A., & Warner, V. (1987). The social adjustment inventory for children and adolescents (SAICA): testing of a new semi-structured interview. *Journal of the American Academy of Child & Adolescent Psychiatry, 26,* 898–911.

Harms, T., Cryer, D., & Clifford, R. M. (1990). *Infant/toddler environment rating scale.* New York, NY: Teachers College Press.

King-Thomas, L. & Hacker, B. (1984). *A therapist's guide to pediatric assessment.* Boston, MA: Little, Brown & Company.

Klein, R., & Bell, B. (1982). *Klein-Bell ADL scale.* Seattle WA: University of Washington, HSCER Distribution.

Knox, S. (1997). Development and current use of the Knox preschool play scale. In L.D. Parham & L.S. Fazio (Eds.), *Play in Occupational Therapy* (pp. 35–51). St. Louis, MO: Mosby–Year Book.

Kunz, K., & Brayman, S. (1999). The comprehensive occupational therapy evaluation. In B. Hemphill-Pearson (Ed.), *Assessments in mental health: An integrative approach* (pp. 259–274), Thorofare, NJ: Slack, Inc.

Law, M., Baptiste, S., Carswell, A., McColl, M., Polatajko, H., & Pollock, N. (1994). *Canadian occupational performance measure.* Toronto, Ontario, CAN: The Canadian Association of Occupational Therapists.

Messick, S. (1995). Validity of psychological assessment: Validation inferences from person's responses and performances as scientific inquiry into score meaning. *American Psychologist, 50(9),* 741–749.

Metro Toronto Community Services Incorporated (1991). Child Care Centre Accessibility Checklist. Toronto, Canada: Author.

Milani-Comparetti, A., & Giodini, E. (1967). Routine developmental examination in neonatal and retarded children. *Developmental Medicine and Child Neurology, 9,* 631–638.

Miller, L. J. (1993). *The first step screening tool*. San Antonio, TX: Psychological Corporation.

Miller, L. J. (1988). *Miller assessment for preschoolers*. San Antonio, TX: Psychological Corporation.

Miller, L. J., & Roid, G. H. (1994). *The T.I.M.E. toddler and infant motor evaluation: A standardized assessment*. Tucson, AZ: Therapy Skill Builders.

Montgomery, P., & Connolly, B. (1987). Norm-references and criterion-referenced tests used in pediatrics and application to task analysis of motor skill. *Physical Therapy, 67*(12), 1873–1876.

Mulligan, S. (2000). Cluster analysis of scores of children on the sensory integration and praxis tests. *Occupational Therapy Journal of Research, 20*(4), 256–262.

Mulligan, S. (1998). Patterns of sensory integration dysfunction: A confirmatory factor analysis. *American Journal of Occupational Therapy, 52*(10), 819–828.

Munro, B. (2001). *Statistical methods for health care research* (4th ed.). Philadelphia, PA: Lippincott Williams & Wilkins.

Murphy, K. R., & Davidshofer, C. O. (1988). *Psychological testing: Principles and applications*. Englewood Cliffs, NJ: Prentice Hall.

Mutti, M., Sterling, H., & Spalding, N. V. (1978). *Quick neurological screening test (qnst)* (Rev. ed.). Los Angeles, CA: Western Psychological Services.

Newborg, J., Stock, J. R., Wnek, L., Guidubaldi, J., & Sviniki, J. (1988). *Battelle developmental inventory, examiner's manual*. Chicago, IL: Riverside.

Piper, M., & Darrah, J. (1994). *Motor assessment of the developing infant*. Philadelphia, PA: W. B. Saunders.

Poresky, R. H. (1987). Environmental assessment index: Reliability, stability and validity of the long and short forms. *Educational and Psychological Measurement, 47*, 969–975.

Provence, S., Erikson, J.,Vater, S., & Palermi, S. (1995). Infant-toddler developmental assessment. Itasca, IL: Riverside Publishing.

Reisman, J. E. (1999). *Minnesota handwriting assessment*. San Antonio, TX: Psychological Corporation.

Russell, D., Rosenbaum, P., Gowland, C., Hardy, S., Lane, M., Plews, N., McGavin, H., Cadman, D., & Jarvis, S. (1993). *Gross motor function measure–revised*. Owen Sound, Ontario, Canada: Pediatric Physiotherapy Services.

Sparrow, S., Balla, D., & Cicchetti, D. (1984). *The Vineland adaptive behavior scales, interview edition: Survey form manual*. Circle Pines, MN: American Guidance Service.

Stern, G. G., Walker, W. J. (1971). *Classroom environment index*. Syracuse, NY: Evaluation Research Associates.

Ulrich, D. (2000). *Test of gross motor development* (2nd Ed.). San Antonio, TX: Psychological Corporation.

Westby, C. E. (1980). Assessment of cognitive and language abilities through play. *Language, Speech, and Hearing Services in Schools, 11,* 154–168.

Yarrow, L. J., Rubenstein, J. L., Pederson, F. A. (1975). *Infant and environment: Early cognitive and motivational development.* New York: Wiley.

Zeitlin, S., Williamson, G. G., & Szczepanski, M. (1988). *Early coping inventory*: Bensenville, IL: Scholastic Testing Service.

SAMPLE REVIEW #1: PEDIATRIC EVALUATION OF DISABILITY INVENTORY (PEDI)

Authors

PEDI Research Group: Haley S, Coster W, Ludlow L, Haltiwanger J, Andrellos P. (Copyright 1992: New England Medical Center Hospital Inc., and PEDI Research Group, Boston, MA.)

Test Description

The PEDI is a functional assessment tool designed for children aged 6 months to 7.5 years (older children can be tested with this tool if their functional abilities fall below the abilities typical of children 7.5 years of age). The PEDI is both a criterion-referenced and a norm-referenced standardized assessment tool, measuring child performance in three main domains: self-care, mobility, and social function. The PEDI is particularly useful for identifying the extent and nature of delays or functional deficits of children with significant motor impairments or a combination of motor and cognitive disabilities. It is less useful for young infants and for children with very mild conditions or for children whose primary disability is psychosocial or behavioral. It is an excellent program evaluation tool and functional outcome measure for pediatric rehabilitation or other intervention programs.

Data may be gathered using a variety of methods, including structured interviews with parents or caregivers and observations of the child by caregivers, therapists, or parents. This test is unique in that there is a scale that measures level of caregiver assistance and a modifications scale to examine the impact of environmental or activity modifications used by the child to complete functional tasks. As a structured parent interview, administration time is approximately 45–60 minutes.

Psychometric Properties

Normative Data

Normative data for the PEDI were gathered from 412 children and families from three New England states. The sample was conveniently selected, and attempts were made to have the sample as representative as possible of the Northeast region of the United States based on estimations derived from 1980 U.S. census data. The following priorities were considered in the selection process: equal age distribution across the age span of 6 months through 7.5 years; equal representation of males and females; race approximating the U.S. population and the region; proportional representation of parent educational levels; and community size (rural versus urban). Overall, the normative data are strong, although the sample is relatively small. Where discrepancies between the sample and the population were identified (e.g., overrepresentation of working mothers), their effects on childrens' functional performance were analyzed, and the demographic variables studied were not found to significantly affect overall PEDI scores. PEDI performance of samples of children from three clinical populations are also included in the manual. Clinical samples included children admitted to a trauma unit (n = 46), 32 children with severe disabilities, and a mixed group of children from a hospital day program with various diagnoses, including cerebral palsy, developmental delay, and traumatic brain injury.

Reliability

Reliability studies measuring internal consistency, inter-interviewer or interrater reliability, and agreement between responses of parents and rehabilitation team members were included in the test manual. Internal consistency measures within the six scales were acceptable, with Cronbach's alpha coefficients ranging from 0.95 to 0.99. Inter-rater reliability for the Caregiver Assistance and Modifications Scales were good, with values ranging from 0.79 to 1.00. Agreement between parents and professionals was adequate, with the exception of scores from the Social Function Scales.

Validity

Construct, content concurrent, and discriminate validity studies are reported in the test manual. The construct of pediatric function for the PEDI was developed from accepted definitions from the World Health Organization. More information on the conceptual model defining pediatric function is provided in the test manual and is available from Coster and Haley (1992). Age-related trends were established, as the mean PEDI scores increased with age, as would be expected. Content validity was addressed extensively throughout the development of the PEDI, and a full chapter in the test manual is devoted to this topic. Review by a panel of experts, evaluation of preliminary research editions, and a combination of statistical techniques, including Rasch scaling and analysis, were conducted to establish the content of the PEDI (see Haley et al., 1991). Concurrent validity was established by correlating scores of children from the normative sample and from clinical samples on the PEDI with scores from the Battelle Developmental Inventory Screening Test and from the Functional Independence Measure for Children , with resultant moderate to high correlations ranging from 0.70 to 0.97. PEDI scores could also discriminate children with known disabilities from those without disabilities.

Practical Considerations

The PEDI is quick (about 30–45minutes) and easy to administer and score, and because it relies on interview techniques, no specialized equipment is necessary. It is relatively inexpensive, costing approximately $90.00, and $125.00 for the optional scoring computer software.

Overall Strengths and Weaknesses

The PEDI is a well-researched tool and an effective measure of rehabilitation outcomes, particularly for children with cerebral palsy and other neuromotor impairments. It is one of the few standardized measures of occupational performance.

Suggested Readings

Feldman, A. B., Haley, S. M., & Coryell, J. (1990). Concurrent and construct validity of the Pediatric Evaluation of Disability Inventory. *Physical Therapy 70*, 602–610.

Haley, S. M., Coster, W., & Faas, R. (1991). A content validity study of the Pediatric Evaluation of Disability Inventory. *Pediatric Physical Therapy, 3*, 177–184.

Nichols, D. S., & Case-Smith, J. (1996). Reliability and validity of the pediatric evaluation of disability inventory. *Pediatric Physical Therapy, 8*, 15–24.

Knox, V. (2000). Clinical review of the pediatric evaluation of disability inventory. *British Journal of Occupational Therapy, 63*, 29–32.

Reid, D. T., Boschen, K., & Wright, V. (1993). Critique of the pediatric evaluation of disability inventory (PEDI). *Physical and Occupational Therapy in Pediatrics, 13*, 57–87.

SAMPLE REVIEW #2: PEABODY DEVELOPMENTAL MOTOR SCALES–2 (PDMS-2)

Author(s)

Folio. R., & Fewell, R. (Copyright 2000, Pro-Ed, Austin TX. 1–800–897–3202)

Test Description

The PDMS-2 is both a norm-referenced and a criteria-referenced standardized assessment tool. It consists of six subtests that measure fine and gross motor performance in children from birth through 6 years of age. Subtests include reflexes (for infants to 12 months of age), stationary gross motor skills, locomotion, object manipulation, grasping, and visual-motor integration. Subtest standard scores and composite standard scores for fine motor, gross motor, and total motor skill are available, as are age-equivalent scores. The test comes with a test kit that includes some (but not all) of the necessary test equipment and supplies, scoring sheets, an examiner's manual, an item administration manual, a motor development chart, and a programming manual and activity cards.

Psychometric Properties

Normative Data

Normative data from 2,003 U.S. children were collected in 1997–1998. Four major U.S. geographic regions were identified as norming sites, and children from 46 states and one Canadian province were included. The normative data were compared with 1997 U.S. Census data and found to be representative of demographic characteristics to describe children younger than 5 years, including geographic area, gender, race, type of residence (rural versus urban), ethnicity, and socioeconomic status. Overall, the normative data are very impressive, including recent data and a large representative sample of typical children. Normative data for children with specific disabilities are not included.

Internal consistency measures using Cronbach's coefficient alphas ranged from 0.84 to 0.98, indicating that test items measuring the same construct (fine and gross motor skills) were strongly associated with one another. Standard errors of measurement for each of the subtests and composite scores by age group are acceptable. Test-retest reliability was evaluated with two groups of children aged 2 through 11 months (n = 20) and 12 to 17 months (n = 30) with acceptable results, with correlation coefficients ranging from 0.73 to 0.96. Interrater reliability for scoring completed protocols has been evaluated, with strong coefficients ranging from 0.96 to 0.98. However, it is believed that discrepancies related to examiner error would more likely occur in the rating of the child's performance on test items rather than during scoring procedures, which has yet to be tested.

Validity

Rationale for the development of test items is described in detail in the manual, with strong theoretical support, and has also been addressed and well researched with the earlier version of the test. Various item analysis techniques were used, including the application of Item Response Theory and logistic regression to analyze differential item functioning, which supported the PDMS-2 content. Age-related trends were established, as the mean PDMS-2 scores increased with age, as would be expected. Confirmatory factor analysis was also used and supported the inclusion of the various subtests within each of the fine and gross motor composites. Concurrent validity was established by correlating PDMS-2 scores of children from the normative sample with their scores on the earlier version of the PDMS-2. Resultant correlations for the fine motor and gross motor composites were strong, 0.84, and 0.91, respectively. PDMS-2 scores also had moderate to strong correlations with scores from the gross and fine motor scales of the Mullen Scales of Early Learning: AGS Edition. PDMS-2 scores could also discriminate children with physical and mental disabilities from those without disabilities.

Practical Considerations: The PDMS-2 is easy to learn, although time and practice are required to become familiar with the administration of the test items. It takes about 60 minutes to administer the entire battery, although the administration process may be broken up if necessary. Space for running, ball throwing, and kicking is necessary. It is relatively expensive, with the test kit costing approximately $525.00.

Overall Strengths and Weaknesses: The PDMS-2 is an excellent tool for measuring overall fine and gross motor skills, although administration time is relatively long. It is easy to learn. It is a well-known test, and although research on the new edition is limited, there an abundance of research on the earlier version.

Suggested Readings

Crowe, T., McClain, C., & Provost, B. (1999). Motor development of Native American children on the Peabody Developmental Motor Scales. *American Journal of Occupational Therapy, 53,* 514–518.

Gebhard, A.R. (1994). Interrater reliability of the Peabody Developmental Motor Scales: fine motor scale. *American Journal of Occupational Therapy, 48,* 976–981.

Russell, D. J. (1994). Test-retest reliability of the fine motor scale of the Peabody Developmental Motor Scales in children with cerebral palsy. *Occupational Therapy Journal of Research, 14,* 178–82.

Tabatabainia, M. M. (1995). Construct validity of the Bruininks-Oseretsky Test of Motor Proficiency and the Peabody Developmental Motor Scales. *Austrialian Occupational Therapy Journal, 42,* 3–13.

Wiart, L., & Darrah, J. (2001). Review of four tests of gross motor development. *Developmental Medicine & Child Neurology , 43,* 279–285.

5
INTERVIEWS AND OBSERVATIONS

INTRODUCTION

This chapter discusses nonstandardized evaluation procedures, including interview techniques and various types of formal and informal observations and procedures. Standardized tests are limited in that they measure performance in very specific areas, and under prescribed rather than naturalistic conditions, with scores being derived from a reference group of individuals or criteria (Cermak, 1989). It is often difficult to know exactly what doing well or poorly on a standardized test really means for an individual's occupational performance unless occupational performance was measured directly. Therefore, conducting nonstandardized procedures as a part of your evaluation is essential. Advantages of using nonstandardized procedures are they tend to be quick and easy to administer, and that they do not require extensive training. Although they are sometimes time consuming, they are inexpensive, noninvasive for the client, and often contextually relevant. They also allow you the flexibility to tailor your evaluation activities to each individual child and family so that you have the opportunity to evaluate important areas that are specifically relevant for individual children and families.

Chapter 5 begins by presenting information about interviews, including strategies and sample interview formats to help you enhance your interview skills. Conducting naturalistic observations in classrooms, during play, and during the performance of functional self-help skills is discussed next. Third, structured observations, including those that can be made during the administration of standardized tests, are discussed, followed by a description of some of the more common formal clinical observation procedures often included as part of pediatric occupational therapy evaluations.

INTERVIEWING

In all areas of occupational therapy practice, evaluations include client interviews. In pediatrics, it is important to interview the child's caregiver or parent(s), the child (depending on the age and maturity of the child), and other important persons in the child's life, such as the child's teacher or child care provider. Interviews provide a unique opportunity to establish rapport with your client and his or her family and to learn about the occupations, roles, and activities they value. Through interviewing, you will also gather vital information about your client's expectations related to your involvement and about his or her priorities, and you will begin to understand how your client sees his or her situation. Interview data are also important because such information can help support and augment data from other sources, such as standardized assessments and observations.

The many different types of interviews range from very informal (lets chat and get to know one another) to very formal and procedural (such as standardized assessment tools that apply interview techniques and consist of a specific set and order of questions). However, there are some general interview techniques that will enhance your effectiveness as an interviewer and that can be applied regardless of the situation and the age of the interviewee. These techniques are discussed further in the following subsections.

Prepare for Your Interviews

To be an effective interviewer, you need to take time to prepare for your interview. It is helpful to set clear goals about

BOX 5-1	COMMON INTERVIEW GOALS

1. To gather relevant medical information, detailed information about the referral concerns, and information about medical and education services the child is receiving or had received in the past.
2. To build a therapeutic alliance and begin to establish rapport and trust.
3. To get to know the child and family better, including their interests and daily life activities.
4. To identify child and family goals, expectations, and priorities.
5. To provide an opportunity to conduct informal observations of clients and environments.
6. To share information about your skills, roles, and services.

what information you want to gather and what you want to accomplish. Examples of goals that can be achieved through client interviews are provided in Box 5-1. In preparing for the interview, draft some questions that you would like to ask and anticipate what questions the interviewee may have for you so you can prepare to respond to their needs. Depending on your situation, there may be sensitive areas you wish to discuss. Anticipate questions that may evoke an emotional response or that may be uncomfortable for you or the interviewee, and think about effective ways you can deal with them.

Create a Comfortable, Relaxed Atmosphere

You will gain the most useful information if you and your clients are relaxed and comfortable during the interview. First, scheduling interviews during times that are convenient and when major distractions are unlikely to occur is vital. The physical environment should be comfortable, including consideration of lighting, temperature, and seating arrangements. In pediatrics you will need to be flexible by conducting caregiver interviews around child schedules and in finding ways to manage the interview when children must be present (see Fig. 5-1). As you begin, always make sure that the interviewee knows why he or she is being interviewed and that he or she can ask questions of

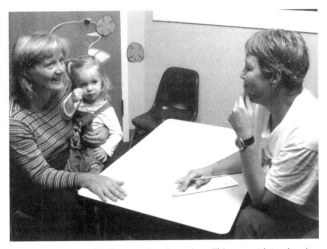

Figure 5-1 Example of a caregiver interview. This parent interview is being conducted with the child present on the parent's lap. It is important to be flexible and for both the interviewer and the interviewee to feel comfortable.

you at any time. Explain your reasons for conducting the interview in language that your interviewee understands. It is important to be aware of and sensitive to the physical and emotional needs of the interviewee. Be aware of your nonverbal language, and constantly be reading and responding appropriately to the nonverbal messages you receive from the interviewee.

Use Strategies to Promote Interaction

The ways in which questions are formulated and asked will affect the amount and quality of information received. Most important, listen, listen, listen, and then listen some more. Building your questions from what your client has just told you is a nice technique that provides the interviewee with a clear message that you care about and are listening carefully to what they are saying. Frequently ask for clarification, or paraphrase what your client has told you, to ensure that you understood what they were trying to tell you. Use open-ended instead of yes/no questions as much as possible because they promote interaction (e.g., "Tell me more about..." and "What would you like me to know about your son?") Although this is sometimes difficult, allow for some silence now and again without being too quick to jump in with a comment or another question. Such pauses provide time for reflection, for you and the interviewee to process what has been said, and to organize your thoughts for the next exchange. Indications that an interview has been effective are that you needed to ask very few questions, your client did most of the talking, the atmosphere was pleasant and comfortable, and the information gained fulfilled your goals.

Structure the Interview With a Beginning, Middle, and End

The interview process should flow smoothly, with a natural beginning, middle, and end. The beginning typically includes introductions, going over the reasons for the interview, and perhaps some "small talk" to ease into the interview. The middle of the interview is the period when most of information is gathered. About 5 to 10 minutes before ending the interview it is important to begin to prepare for the end of the interview. This is accomplished by first letting the interviewee know that time is almost up so he or she has an opportunity to ask any final questions of you or to share any information that was left out earlier. It is important to have time to thank the interviewee, to share how the information will be used, and to describe the next step in the evaluation process.

Although interviews are conducted with caregivers for various reasons, the most important reason is to give the parent an opportunity to tell his or her story so that you can begin to understand who he or she is and who the child is. You will always customize your interview style with caregivers to fit their individual personality and needs and so that you can achieve the goals that you set for the interview. Sample questions used in an initial caregiver interview are provided in Box 5-2 to help guide your interviews and gather relevant information useful for intervention planning.

BOX 5-2	SAMPLE QUESTIONS USED IN AN INITIAL INTERVIEW WITH J.'S MOTHER

Gather Demographic Information:

Child and parents' names, address, telephone number, and child's date of birth should be gathered ahead of time. Who lives in the home? What are the ages of the other children? What is the easiest way for me to contact you? Who is J.'s primary physician? For billing purposes, I need to gather information about your health insurance.

Gather Medical History Information:

I would like find out a little more about J.'s early history. Did you (if interviewing the mother) have any complications with your pregnancy or delivery with J.? How long did you spend in the hospital? At what age did J. learn to sit up? Smile? Crawl? Walk? Has J. had any major illnesses or hospitalizations? (If yes, can you tell me a little bit about what happened?) Does he have a history of allergies or ear infections? What have been the results of eyesight and hearing tests? Does J. take any medications? Tell me what led you to seek out occupational therapy services for J. What have you learned about J.'s development from other professionals who have worked with or evaluated J.? Is there anything else about his medical history or current condition you think I should know?

Gather Information About the Child and His or Her Family:

Tell me about J. How does J. typically spend his time? What does J. like to do at home? At school? Does J. have any particular fears or dislikes? Does J. participate in extracurricular activities? (If yes, tell me about these activities.) What kinds of things do you do as a family? What responsibilities do J. and his siblings have around the house? Do you have neighbors, friends, or relatives that you can depend on to help you if needed? What do you and your husband do for work? Tell me about J.'s child care situation? What is J. really good at?

Gather Information About the Child's School Program and Other Services:

Tell me about J.'s school program. What is his teacher like? How is his day structured at school and what kinds of skills is he currently working on? What is important to you regarding his school program? How is he doing at school? Tell me about the other services he is currently receiving.

Identify Child and Family Priorities and Goals:

What are the skills or areas that you would like us to address most in occupational therapy? In terms of J.'s development and skills, what are your priorities? In developing a program for you and J., is there anything else that you think I should know about J. or your family that would help me tailor your program to meet your goals and expectations?

Considerations for Conducting Interviews With Children

A few important considerations must be kept in mind when you are interviewing children. First, you must acknowledge the developmental level of the child you are interviewing. The ability of a child to express his or her thoughts and feelings depends on various language and other cognitive prerequisite skills. For example, typically, children younger than 8 years will describe themselves only in terms of observable traits and not by internal characteristics (Stone and Lemanek, 1990). The accuracy of information reported by children of this age is also questionable. Therefore, interviews with children younger than 8 years generally should be conducted mainly to establish rapport and to get to know their likes and dislikes. Several clinical observations can also be made during an interview with a child, such as his or her ability to communicate, interact, and follow directions and his or her affect and activity level.

As the capacity for abstract thinking becomes more sophisticated, young adolescents are more able to reliably answer questions. They probably have the capacity for self-reflection and can begin to describe their feelings, behaviors, and skills in relation to those of their peers and can comment on how others view their behavior. Therefore, the amount of information that can be obtained through interviews with older children and adolescents is far greater than what can be obtained through interviews with young children.

STANDARDIZED ASSESSMENT TOOLS USING STRUCTURED INTERVIEWS

Most standardized occupational therapy interview assessments have been designed for adults, although a few are available specifically for pediatric practice. Some of the more commonly used tools include the Canadian Occupational Performance Measure (Law et al., 1994), the Pediatric Evaluation of Disability Inventory (Haley et al., 1992), the Sensory Profile (Dunn, 1999), and the Adolescent Role Assessment (Black, 1976). Although the Pediatric Evaluation of Disability Inventory and the Sensory Profile can be completed by the caregiver independently (caregiver completes assessment forms without the therapist present), it is nice to take the time to conduct the assessment as an interview. This ensures that the caregiver understands the questions and provides an opportunity for the interviewee to elaborate on the areas included on the assessment. This dialog provides for more detailed and richer information than can be gained from the checked responses on the testing booklets alone. More information about these assessment tools is included in the tables describing standardized assessment tools in Chapter 4.

CONDUCTING OBSERVATIONS

Your structured and unstructured observations often will be the most valuable sources of information gathered throughout the evaluation process. Your observations are simply defined as what you see. Although this sounds straightforward, it is important and sometimes challenging to distinguish mere observations from your interpretations of the behaviors observed. For example, suppose that during a 30-minute evaluation session a 6-year-old child was observed to cry briefly on separation from her mother and then to have very flat affect (little facial expression) for the rest of the session. She refused to engage in 8 of 10 activities presented to her, she answered questions using only one-word answers, and she initiated no conversation. Overall, she seemed very sad, lethargic, withdrawn, and somewhat noncompliant.

The behaviors that were observed included crying, flat affect, little use of language, refusing to engage in most activities presented to her, and having a low activity level. These observations are clear and quite undisputable. However, these observed behaviors may be interpreted in various different ways. For example, one may conclude that she is demonstrating symptoms of depression or has feelings of sadness. Another interpretation may be that she is shy and has trouble relating to strangers. And yet another is that she simply did not want to be evaluated and was therefore acting defiant. This example demonstrates that there are many ways that observed behavior can be interpreted and why it is so important during the evaluation process, particularly in your report writing, that you explicitly differentiate between what it is you observed (exactly what you saw) and how you interpreted your observations.

Observations can be recorded in various ways, and, whenever possible, it is important to document observations in an objective rather than a subjective manner. There are three main ways that observations can be recorded. First, you may use narrative description, which provides a detailed account of and qualitative information about the behaviors observed. Second, when you are looking for specific behaviors, you could record the rate of the behavior by using either a frequency count (the number of times the behavior occurred in a given period) or duration recording (the length of time the behavior occurred). To perform a frequency count or duration recording, it is important that the behavior to be observed is operationally defined so that it is clear what the behavior is, when it begins, and when it no longer meets the criteria for being present. A third way to record observations is to record the behavior on a self-designed data recording form that may be in the form of a checklist or rating scale. Often such forms also include space for writing narrative descriptions.

For the purposes of this book, observations have been classified into three main categories: naturalistic observations; structured observations, including those that can be made during the administration of standardized tests; and formal clinical observation procedures. Each category is discussed in more detail in the following subsections.

Naturalistic Observations

Naturalistic observations are those that take place in the context of the child's regular activities and environment. True naturalistic observations also require that you as the observer be as unobtrusive as possible so that your presence does not affect the way the child or anyone else in the environment would usually perform. Three common types of naturalistic observations conducted by pediatric occupational therapists are classroom observations; observations of play in the home, school, and child-care environments; and observations of children performing functional tasks such as feeding, dressing, and household and vocational tasks.

Classroom Observations
Classroom observations are a part of most school-based occupational therapy evaluations. Such evaluations are

provided under the Individuals With Disabilities Act and therefore must follow the regulations set forth in this legislation. Seeing first hand how the child's classroom is run, what the child's curriculum entails, and how the child functions in the classroom provides valuable information for program planning and assists in determining the educational relevance or impact a child's deficits have on his or her ability to be successful in the classroom.

In preparing for a classroom observation, it is important to speak with the child's parent(s) and teacher to discuss any concerns or questions they have regarding the child's school performance and to find out what they think is important for you to observe. Once the behaviors in question have been identified, you and the teacher can decide together when the most appropriate time and place to conduct the observation would be. For example, if the child has fine motor and attention difficulties, it might be most useful to observe the child during a sit-down art activity or a writing task.

Self-designed checklists and rating scales may be developed and used to help structure and document classroom observations. An example of a self-designed classroom observation form is provided in Figure 5-2. Although the school-related skills and areas that you will be interested in observing will vary greatly depending on the age or grade of the child and on the child's needs, examples of typical skills and areas that occupational therapists are asked to assess are included in this observation form.

Observations of Play

Although a few standardized assessment tools are available for evaluating play (see Chapter 4), you may choose to observe a child's play more informally in the context of regular play situations at home, at school, or in the child-care setting. Play is complex, and, as the primary occupation of children, it is of great interest to occupational therapists. Play is the means by which infants and young children learn, have fun, and interact. Evaluations of play should include gathering information about a child's ability to engage in meaningful play, their playfulness, play preferences, and social play behaviors and skills. Also, by conducting observations of children's play, information can often be gathered on various underlying skill areas and client factors. For example, you can learn a great deal about a child's fine and gross motor skills, balance and postural control, social communication, and cognitive skills (e.g., knowledge of shapes, colors, and size concepts) by watching them play. It is also important to observe psychosocial skills and behaviors, such as activity level, affect, ability to express emotions, and emotional stability. Social interaction patterns between the child and the caregiver and among peers can also be evaluated through unstructured play observations.

Reviewing the typical play behaviors and skills exhibited by children of various ages and developmental levels will help you identify the specific behaviors to look for when evaluating individual clients (see Chapter 3). A guide to help you structure and gather important information about a child's play preferences, use of materials, social play behaviors, adaptability, and other psycho-emotional factors is provided in Box 5-3. Examples of play observations are provided in Figures 5-3 and 5-4.

When conducting evaluations of the play or leisure skills and interests of older school-aged children and adolescents, it may be most useful to observe them with their peers during a group recreational or leisure activity. In addition, much can be learned about their use of leisure time, their interests, and their social skills by interviewing them and their caregivers.

Observations of Functional Activities

Information about a child's ability to perform basic self-help skills such as feeding and toileting and to participate in household tasks and vocational activities is often gathered through parent report. Standardized assessment tools that use an interview or observation format, such as the Pediatric Evaluation of Disability Inventory (Haley et al., 1992), and observations of the child performing the functional activities of concern or interest, provide the most objective and detailed information. Direct observations are particularly useful if the child can be assessed during the times the activities naturally occur and in the settings where they are typically performed. Conducting naturalistic observations of children performing functional skills allows you to formulate a comprehensive understanding of

(*Text continued on page 214*)

School Observation Form

Student Name _____ DOB _____ Grade _____ Teacher _____

Special Education Services: _____

Teacher and Parent Concerns: _____

Date of Observation: _____

Activities Observed: _____

Classroom Environment: (desk arrangements, traffic patterns, work areas, auditory and visual stimuli, etc.)

Sensory Motor Observations

Skill	Problem	Not a Problem	Comments
Sitting			
Functional mobility			
Fine motor, handwriting			
Gross motor coordination			
Strength and endurance			
Visual processing			

Performance of Classroom Activities and Behavior

Skill	Problem	Not a Problem	Comments
Attention/activity level			
Task completion			
Works independently			
Follows directions			
Communication skills			
Self-care skills: snack and lunch, toileting, dressing, managing belongings			
Use of classroom materials			
Accesses playground, lunchroom, hallways, lockers			
Transitions smoothly between activities			
Interacts well with peers			
Respects teacher			

Curriculum Modifications:
Summary:

Figure 5–2. Sample classroom observation form.

BOX 5-3   GUIDE FOR CONDUCTING OBSERVATIONS
OF PLAY

Document the Child's Play Preferences:

What does the child seem to like? Dislike? What does the child spend
the most time doing during play? What characterizes the types of
toys or activities the child prefers? Does the child spend more time in
sedentary or active play? What are the specific sensory features of the
toys the child chooses? Does the child prefer unstructured and creative play or play that is structured and has rules? Does the child tend
to play alone or to seek out others during free play? What roles does
the child assume during play (observer, leader, or follower)?

**Document the Ways in Which the Child Uses Materials and
Play Equipment:**

Does the child use toys in the ways in which they were intended to
be used? How many different ways does the child use the same play
materials? Are materials used in a perseverative fashion? How competent is the child in manipulating materials and toys (comment on
dexterity, grasp and release patterns, fine motor coordination). Does
the child seem to have the ability to move and the strength and coordination to engage in age appropriate gross motor play? What does
the child do well? Does the child initiate play? For how long does the
child engage in the same play activity? Is the child curious and
excited about exploring novel objects and play situations?

Document the Child's Social Play Behaviors:

Does the child tend to play alone or with others? Is the child comfortable with parallel play? Does the child interact verbally and non-
verbally with peers? Does the child share materials? Is the child willing to take turns? Does the child engage others actively in play
situations? Is the child willing and able to adapt play situations to
accommodate others? How does the child use language and other
means to communicate during play? How well does the child communicate his or her wants and needs during play? Does the child
seem to enjoy playing with others or alone?

**Document Any Psychosocial and Emotional Factors Observed
During Play:**

Does the child transition easily to and from different play activities?
How long does the child typically stay with or attend to a specific
play activity? Does the child engage in an approach-avoidance
behavior (goes to an activity briefly like he or she wants to participate but then leaves the activity)? What is the child's affect and ability to express emotion? What emotions seem to be expressed by
facial expressions and behaviors? Does the child seem interested in
the environment and play opportunities? Engaged? Bored? Aggressive? Passive? Cooperative? Does the child persist when challenged
or become easily frustrated and give up when challenged?

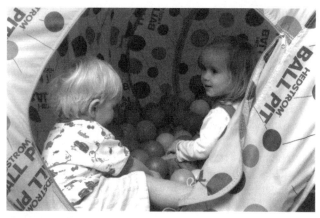

Figure 5-3 Observations during play. These two children, 25 and 21 months of age, are observed playing in a tunnel filled with small plastic balls. During play, these children look frequently at one another and are comfortable next to each other but do not engage in social play. They seem to enjoy playing in the tunnel of balls, tolerating the tactile, visual, and auditory stimuli it provides without difficulty. They explore the balls, move well in the tunnel by crawling, and are both stable in sitting to free their hands to explore and toss the balls. They demonstrate the ability to grasp and release the balls, although they show little throwing accuracy. The older child identifies some of the colors, and the younger child frequently says the word "ball."

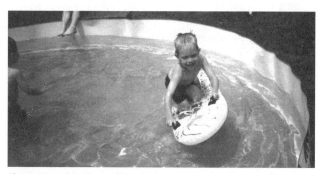

Figure 5-4 This 4-year-old is playing with friends in a backyard pool. He demonstrates the ability to motor plan a novel task by successfully climbing onto the raft and positioning himself for a ride. He is able to stabilize himself in a 4-point position, and he demonstrates effective body and head righting reactions to maintain his balance and avoid tipping. His hands grip the handles tightly, and he demonstrates adequate cocontraction at the shoulders and mobilization to accommodate the movement of the raft. He enjoys this unpredictable movement experience. He engages in parallel play by being comfortable being in close proximity with other children in the pool and doing his own thing.

the child's strengths and challenges and of the techniques and strategies used to accomplish the tasks. The influences of the environment and the demands of each task observed can also be determined, which is helpful for intervention planning. Depending on your work setting and client population (age, diagnosis, etc.), you will want to observe different types of functional skills. Consideration of the child's occupational profile, which is established early in the evaluation process, will assist you in selecting the functional tasks that would be most important for you to observe in individual clients. Tables 5-1 and 5-2 list some of the common functional tasks that occupational therapists observe as part of comprehensive evaluations of children of different ages.

When evaluating functional tasks, it is important to include the following:

1. A description of the context in which the activity takes place, including environmental factors and task demands.
2. The child's level of independence and the level and type of assistance required for the child to complete the activity (common terminology used by occupational therapists to describe levels of assistance was provided in Chapter 2).
3. Any special techniques, compensatory strategies, and adaptive equipment used to complete the task.
4. A description of how the child completes the activity, including positions and movements used and kinds of errors made.
5. Any underlying deficits or client factors (medical, sensory, motor, cognitive, psychosocial, and emotional) that seem to be interfering with the child's ability to perform the task efficiently and safely.

Structured Observations

When you do not have the time or opportunity to observe your client performing in context the functional skills or activities that have been identified as important and challenging, it may be necessary to set up an evaluation situation in which the child is asked to perform the functional skills out of context. In general, observing children in their natural context is a bit risky because child behavior is more unpredictable than adult behavior and you may not get the

TABLE 5-1	SUGGESTED FUNCTIONAL ACTIVITIES TO OBSERVE WITH CHILDREN 0–5 YEARS OF AGE
Age	**Suggested Functional Activities**
Birth to 1 year	Observe play skills and caregiver-infant interaction patterns during play and during caregiving activities; note the infant's ability to communicate needs and wants through gestures, facial expressions, and verbalizations; note attachment behaviors and ability to self-regulate, including maintaining active, alert states and ability to self-calm; observe caretaking activities, including feeding, bathing, and dressing, and the child's mobility and functional use of the upper extremities for play
1–3 years	Observe play skills and caregiver-infant interaction patterns during play and caregiving activities; note the child's ability to communicate needs and wants through language and nonverbal means and his or her ability to follow simple directions; observe the child's ability to play and interact with peers and to play independently; note attachment behaviors and ability to separate from parent; observe feeding, dressing, toileting, mobility, and functional use of the upper extremities for play
3–5 years	Observe play skills and caregiver-infant interaction patterns during play and caregiving activities; note the child's ability to use language and other means to communicate needs and wants, make comments, ask questions, share information, and follow directions; observe the child's ability to play and interact with peers and to play independently; note attachment behaviors and ability to separate from parent and the development of self-control; observe feeding, dressing, bathing, toileting, mobility, and functional use of the upper extremities for play; observe the child's ability to participate in typical preschool activities, such as sitting quietly in a group for 10–15 min, following directions, and following a classroom routine; safety judgment on the playground; observe use of assistive technology if applicable

TABLE 5-2	SUGGESTED FUNCTIONAL ACTIVITIES TO OBSERVE WITH CHILDREN 5–18 YEARS OF AGE	
Age	**School Settings**	**Hospital Settings**
School-aged children	Observe written, verbal, and nonverbal communication skills; self-feeding and lunchroom independence; toileting and simple age-appropriate grooming activities; functional mobility, including classroom seating, movement, and safety within school environments and with bus transportation; manipulation of educational materials; participation in classroom activities and specialized classes such as art, music, and physical education; computer use and use of assistive technology, if necessary; peer interactions; ability to attend and work independently, complete assignments, and participate in small and large group work with peers; for older children, observe basic community living and prevocational activities	Observe verbal and nonverbal communication skills; self-feeding; bathing, grooming, toileting, and functional mobility, including bed mobility, transfers, and walking; computer use and use of assistive technology, if applicable; ability to participate in play or leisure skills and to interact with peers; for older children, observe basic community living and prevocational activities

opportunity to see exactly what you are looking for. Setting up evaluation situations and activities deliberately and purposely increases the probability that you will observe the behaviors and skills of most interest. The development and setup of informal, meaningful evaluation activities involves applying your knowledge of the child's occupational profile, common sense, and a bit of creativity. Specific equipment, materials, or space may also be necessary. Examples of setting up structured observations for evaluating specific areas or skills are provided in Boxes 5-4 and 5-5.

Clinical observations can also be made during the administration of standardized tests. For example, dur-

---

BOX 5-4   SETTING UP STRUCTURED OBSERVATIONS OF
GROSS MOTOR SKILLS

Clinic Setting:

Plan a 10-min play situation that limits the child's play choices to
gross motor activities. For example, set up an obstacle course with
a climbing apparatus, a tunnel, and a balance beam. Depending on
the age of the child, have large therapy balls, a suspended platform
swing, a rocker board, a riding toy, balls of various sizes, and a mini-
trampoline available as play choices. For an infant or child with significant neuromotor deficits, you may purposefully place the child in
various positions to examine sitting posture and balance, postural
control, movement, and ability to play in prone and in supine. If you
suspect that a child is overly sensitive to or fearful of movement
(posturally insecure), gently place him or her on a therapy ball in the
sitting position or on a suspended swing and observe the child's
reaction to having his or her feet off of the ground. Ask the child to
perform some age-appropriate gross motor skills (e.g., sit-ups,
climbing stairs, jumping rope, running, push-ups, hopping, skip-
ping, jumping jacks, and playing catch).

Home Setting:

Many of the ideas listed for the clinical setting can be implemented
in the home or in a backyard. Whenever possible, observe activities
that the child participates in, such as watching the child ride his own
riding toys or play on his backyard swing set.

---

ing administration of a test of visual-motor integration,
such as the Beery-Buktenika Developmental Test of
Visual-Motor Integration (Beery, 1997), which is a
design copy test, you can take note of the child's sitting
posture, ability to follow directions, and attend. Motor
planning and sequencing skills; basic pencil skills,
including grasp patterns; hand preference; pencil pressure; and coordination of the pencil during a drawing
task can also be observed. Depending on the age of the
child, following test administration, you may also wish
to have the child do a short writing sample, such as
printing his or her name, address, and telephone number. In addition to gaining a standardized score of visual
motor skill you will gain insight into some functional
handwriting skills and fine motor skills.

The options for developing structured observations are
limitless. Therefore, it is important that you are very delib-

---

BOX 5-5   STRUCTURED OBSERVATIONS OF PLAY
SPECIFICALLY FOR CHILDREN WITH SUSPECTED
PERVASIVE DEVELOPMENTAL DISORDERS (PDDS)

Clinic, Home, or Preschool Setting:

If one of your evaluation goals is to help determine whether a child
fits the diagnostic criteria for a PDD such as autism, play observations that would increase the probability of observing the kinds of
behaviors that characterize children with autistic spectrum disorders
are helpful. These behaviors include perseverative play; difficulty
transitioning to and from different play materials and play scenarios;
atypical or little use of language; sensory processing differences,
including hypersensitivities or hyposensitivities; and difficulty with
social play, with a preference for solitary play. To help structure your
observations, keep these characteristics in mind and select sensory-
based toys with enticing visual and auditory stimuli and some imag-
inative/pretend toys like a tea set or play farm, and set up turn-tak-
ing games that encourage social interaction. Set up play themes or
materials that the child has a tendency to overfocus on, and ask the
child to transition to and from different activities. Play observations
should include some unstructured, solitary play time and play with
caregivers, peers, and siblings when possible as well as with you.
Opportunities should be provided for the child to assume different
roles (leader and follower), use language, request desired objects,
and interact with others during play.

---

erate in your selection of evaluation activities and that you
set up situations most likely to yield the kinds of observation data that you are looking for. It is important to conduct your evaluation efficiently and to avoid duplication of
data obtained through standardized testing or gathered by
other team members. Other examples of structured observations that can be conducted to evaluate specific child
factors/performance components are given in many of the
tables in Chapter 2. To assist you in writing up your observations, a list of terminology describing movement and
positions and other motor behaviors is given in Table 5-3.

Formal Clinical Observations and Procedures

Formal clinical observations are those that have specific
directions for administration, although they are not performed as part of any specific standardized assessment

TABLE 5-3	TERMINOLOGY USED TO DESCRIBE MOTOR BEHAVIOR AND TO DOCUMENT OBSERVATIONS

Type of Motor Behavior	Common Terminology
Postural control and quality of movement	Head and trunk control; proximal stability at the shoulder and pelvic girdle; weight bearing and base of support; weight shifting, muscle elongation, trunk rotation, body and head righting; random movements, spontaneous movements, purposeful or volitional movement; bilateral movement, symmetry, asymmetry, influence of gravity, antigravity movement; motor coordination terms, including fine and gross motor control, smooth, tremulous; muscle tone descriptors, including hypotonic, flaccid, hypertonic, and rigid
Various positions	Prone, supine, sitting, supported sitting, W-sit, ring sit, long sitting, kneeling, half kneeling, quadruped/crawling or 4-point position, standing, supported standing, anterior or posterior pelvic tilt, lordotic, kyphotic, upright, slouched or flexed forward, midline, prone extension, supine flexion, and sidelying
Direction of movement	Flexion, extension, abduction, adduction, rotation, lateral flexion of the trunk, trunk rotation, internal and external rotation, supination, pronation, dorsiflexion, plantar flexion, inversion, eversion, shoulder retraction, shoulder protraction, and elevation

Although these terms are commonly used by medical professionals, many are not typically used or understood by nonmedical individuals.

tool. Pediatric occupational therapists often use formal procedures to assess underlying sensory motor and postural skills. Although some standardized assessments include test items for this purpose, such as items to measure automatic reactions, reflex behavior, and muscle tone, often these neuromotor components are evaluated separately from a standardized test. Wilson et al. (2000), however, developed a standardized test titled the COMPS—Clinical Observations of Motor and Postural Skills—that provides specific instructions and normative data on many of the more common procedures used by occupational therapists, which are presented later herein.

It is important to realize that many of the clinical observation procedures included in this chapter have not been validated adequately through research, and, for many, the administration procedures used by therapists may vary somewhat (see Dunn, 1981; Gregory-Flock and Yerxa, 1984; Haley, 1987; Harris et al., 1984; Wilson et al., 2000). Therefore, findings from these observations must be interpreted by applying the available research and must be used cautiously alongside your other observations and clinical judgment, the results of standardized tests, and information gathered from medical record reviews and interviews. If you decide to use these observations, it is suggested that you review relevant research associated with each one to ensure that you are interpreting the behaviors that you observe appropriately. When conducting neuromotor and sensory integration clinical observations and procedures, it is important to look for asymmetries or differences in the left versus the right side of the body, so many of these procedures should be performed on both sides of the body. Because primitive reflex patterns and righting and automatic reactions were covered in Chapter 3, they are not included with the observations presented later herein.

Formal Clinical Observations of Neuromotor, Musculoskeletal, and Sensory Integration Functions

Muscle tone: amount of muscle contraction or tension of a muscle at rest

1. Sitting opposite the child, ask him or her to extend arms with forearms supinated, and place wrist flexors on stretch; observe for hyperextensibility in the elbows and wrist, which is an indication of low tone.
2. Examine the amount of resistance during passive movement of the limbs. For example, with the child in supine, move the lower limbs in abduction with knees flexed; move the foot in ankle plantar and dorsiflexion; move the upper extremities in elbow flexion and extension, and shoulder flexion and extension. Little to no resistance is evidence of low tone, and moderate to high resistance is indicative of high tone.

3. Palpate the muscle bellies at rest (e.g., biceps, gastrocnemius); the muscle bellies are soft when muscle tone is low and firm when muscle tone is high.

Supine flexion. Place the child in supine, with arms crossed on the chest, and with the neck, hips, and knees flexed (demonstrate as needed); time how long the child can assume the position; determine whether the child can maintain the position with gentle resistance applied to the head and knees.

Prone extension. Place the child in prone with shoulders abducted and elbows flexed, legs extended with knees off of the floor; demonstrate if needed; time how long the child can assume the position (norms available from Gregory-Flock and Yerxa, 1984; Wilson et al., 2000). The child in Figure 5-5 is experiencing some difficulty assuming the correct posture because he cannot lift his knees off of the floor.

Cocontraction. Cocontraction is the ability of opposing muscle groups to contract at the same time, providing stability around a joint. With the child sitting in a chair across from you, with back unsupported, the child is asked to grab onto your thumbs (put your arms forward with thumbs up). Then, ask the child to stay as still as possible and not to let you push or pull him or her. Allow the child

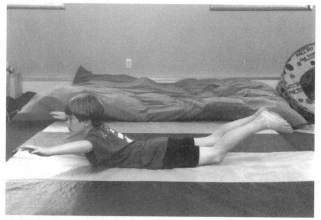

Figure 5-5 Assessment of prone extension.

some elbow flexion, and give the child a chance to build some muscle tone. Then, push and pull in an arc-type motion, up and toward the child and down and away from the child. Do not let the child lock elbows; if the child has good cocontraction, he or she should be able stay relatively still.

Visual pursuits. Sit facing the child. Ask the child to keep his or her head still while allowing his or her eyes to move. Move a pencil or penlight horizontally, vertically, and then diagonally about 8 to 10 inches from the child's eyes; check for quick localization by asking the child to look at the object while you move it quickly in different planes; observe for smoothness of eye movement versus jerky or inaccurate movements, midline jerk, and the child's ability to separate eye movements from head movements (see Fig. 5-6).

Muscle strength

1. Manual muscle testing procedures: To perform manual muscle testing, you must know the muscles of the body and their functions, anatomic positions and direction of the muscle fibers, and angle of pull of the joints. Muscle testing cannot be conducted with children who have abnormal muscle tone. Assignment of a muscle grade depends on clinical judgment, knowl-

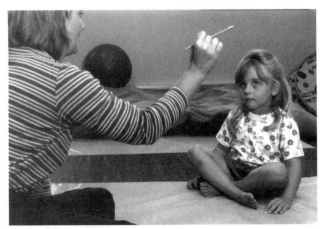

Figure 5-6 Assessment of visual pursuits.

edge, and examiner experience. The grading system used goes from 0 to 5, with low grades representing weakness, and is based on how well the child moves the limb against gravity and by the amount of resistance the individual can endure. Formal manual muscle testing of specific muscles is rarely done with young children because of difficulties with child compliance and understanding of what is required. Specific procedures can be found in numerous other sources and are not included herein (see Neistadt, 2000; Trombly, 1995; Simmonds, 1997).

2. Sit-ups and push-ups: Ask the child to perform as many sit-ups as he or she can in 1 minute and record the number; ask the child to perform as many push-ups as possible in 1 minute and record the number (children 7 years of age and younger and girls can do push-ups from the knees).

Motor coordination

1. Rapid alternating movements: Child and examiner are sitting facing one another, with arms flexed, resting on laps. You demonstrate rapid supination and pronation (slapping thighs gently), first with one hand, then the other hand, then with both hands together. Instruct the child to do it fast, and count the number of times the palms slap the thighs in 10 seconds (should be around 10 times); observe coordination, smoothness of movements, and right-left differences.

2. Thumb-finger touching (see Fig. 5-7): Ask the child, after demonstration, to touch his or her thumb with each finger in sequence from the index to the little finger and then back in sequence to the index finger, repeating several times. First start with one hand, then the other hand, and then both hands simultaneously. Then ask the child to perform the same task with his or her eyes closed. Look for associated reactions, asymmetries, speed and smoothness of movement, and degree of visual input the child requires to complete the task. The child in Figure 5-7 can replicate the movement, although her movements are very slow and deliberate, and some associated movements are noted with the left hand.

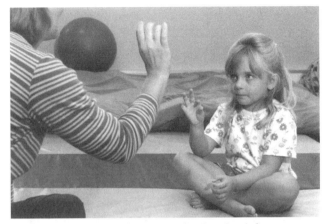

Figure 5-7 Assessment of motor coordination: thumb-finger touching.

SUMMARY

Nonstandardized evaluation procedures, including interviews and observations, were covered in this chapter. Information gained from informal and formal observations and through interviews, particularly with caregivers, may be the most valuable evaluation data you gather throughout the evaluation process. This is particularly true for children who are difficult to test using standardized instruments and for those with severe or profound disabilities, for whom few standardized assessment tools are available. Observing clients perform the activities that they typically do everyday, in their natural contexts, is one of the most exciting, content-rich tools that you can use. Information gained from such naturalistic observations helps you understand what your clients do and how children and families engage in their daily occupations. It is, however, important to consider the limitations of their use, namely, the subjectivity and bias that affect your interpretations and the lack of reliability and validity data supporting the conclusions you draw from nonstandardized procedures. Nonetheless, such informal procedures provide you with the flexibility to individualize your evaluation plan for each child, helping to maximize efficiency and to ensure that you gather evaluation data that are most helpful to you and your clients.

As you gain clinical experience by applying these and other nonstandardized procedures with numerous children and their families, you will become more and more familiar with what you can expect to see from children of various ages and with certain types of disabilities. Although all children must be viewed as individuals, there are some common behaviors that can be predicted based on the ways in which certain types of children typically respond in similar situations. Over time, differences in behavior among children will become more obvious, and your accuracy and confidence in making interpretations of the behaviors you see will grow.

References

Beery, K. (1997). *Beery-Buktenica developmental test of visual-motor integration (VMI)* (4th ed.). Parsippany, NJ: Modern Curriculum Press.

Black, M. (1976). Adolescent role assessment. *American Journal of Occupational Therapy 30,* 73–79.

Cermak, S. (1989). Norms and scores. *Physical and Occupational Therapy in Pediatrics, 9*(1), 91–123.

Dunn, W. (1981). *A guide to testing clinical observations in kindergartners.* Rockvill, MD: American Occupational Therapy Association.

Dunn, W. (1999). *Sensory profile, user's manual.* San Antonio, TX: Psychological Corp.

Gregory-Flock, J.L., & Yerxa, E.J. (1984). Standardization of the prone extension postural test on children ages 4 through 8. *American Journal of Occupational Therapy, 38,* 187–194.

Haley, S.M. (1987). Sequence of development of postural reactions by infants with Down's syndrome. *Developmental and Child Neurology, 29,* 674–679.

Haley, S., Coster, W., Ludlow, L., Haltiwanger, J., & Andrellos, P. (1992). *Pediatric evaluation of disability inventory.* San Antonio, TX: Psychological Corp.

Harris, S., Swanson, M.W., & Chandler, L. (1984). Predictive validity of the movement assessment for infants. *Journal of Behavioral Pediatrics, 5,* 336–342.

Law, M., Baptiste, S., Carswell, A., McColl, M., Polatajko, H., & Pollock, N. (1994). *Canadian occupational performance measure.* Toronto, Ontario, CAN: The Canadian Association of Occupational Therapists.

Neistadt, M. (2000). *Occupational therapy evaluation for adults: A pocket guide*. Philadelphia, PA: Lippincott Williams & Wilkins.

Simmonds, M. (1997). Muscle Strength. In J. Van Deusen & D. Brunts Eds. *Assessment in occupational therapy and physical therapy* (pp. 27–48). Philadelphia, PA: W.B. Saunders Company.

Stone, W.L., & Lemanek, K.L. (1990). Developmental issues in children's self-reports. In A.M. LaGreca (Ed.), *Through the eyes of the child. Obtaining self-reports from children and adolescents* (pp. 18–55). Boston, MA: Allyn & Bacon.

Trombly, C.A. (1995). Evaluation of biomechanical and physiological aspects of motor performance. In C.A. Trombly (Ed.), *Occupational therapy for physical dysfunction* (4th ed. pp. 73–156). Baltimore: Williams & Wilkins.

Wilson, B.N., Pollock, N., Kaplan, B.J., & Law, M. (2000). *Clinical observations of motor and postural Skills (COMPS)*. Framingham, MA: Therapro.

6
WORKING AS A MEMBER OF A TEAM

INTRODUCTION

It is rare that occupational therapists work independently in pediatrics. The evaluation process more often is conducted collaboratively with professionals from various disciplines. Children with disabilities are complex. They benefit most from a holistic approach guided by individuals from different disciplines that bring their own skills and areas of expertise to the evaluation process and to the child's program. Federal legislation requires that infants and children in early intervention and those receiving services through their educational programs be evaluated by a team of professionals representing multiple disciplines (Individuals With Disabilities Education Act [IDEA], 1997).

Groups of professionals organize themselves to form teams, and there are three main types of team models: **multidisciplinary, interdisciplinary**, and **transdisciplinary** (McCormack and Goldman, 1979; Case-Smith, 2001). These team models differ from one another primarily with respect to the extent or depth of collaboration among the team members and the degree to which they share roles. Regardless of the type of team you find yourself on, there are several competencies and personal qualities that will assist you in functioning well as a team member. Such competencies also allow teams as a whole to function well and help create productive, fulfilling, and pleasant working environments. **Team member competencies** are described in detail in the literature on team building and effective communication, organizational behavior, and group process. Some of the most important competencies that will allow you to be an effective team member are presented in Box 6-1.

This chapter begins with a description of the **discipline-specific roles** of professionals with whom occupational therapists commonly work in pediatrics. The members of a child's team largely depends on the work setting (medical versus educational), the type and severity of the child's disability, the child's age, and support networks (Case-Smith, 2001). A description of the three types of team models—multidisciplinary, interdisciplinary, and transdisciplinary—follows. The last part of this chapter presents information describing some assessment tools and evaluation techniques that you may find useful for conducting **collaborative evaluations**. An interdisciplinary team evaluation of a child in early intervention; an educational, trans-

BOX 6-1	COMPETENCIES FOR BEING AN EFFECTIVE TEAM MEMBER

Consistency with your discipline-specific roles and philosophy

The ability to be flexible and open to new ideas

Clear nonverbal and verbal communication; asking for clarification as needed

Effective interpersonal and communication skills

Being respectful of others and being a good listener

Leadership skills, including being goal directed, visionary, and organized

Willingness and ability to share your knowledge, skills, and resources

Being committed to fulfilling your responsibility for meeting team goals

The ability to effectively receive and apply feedback about your performance as a team member

The ability to facilitate and participate in effective group problem solving and decision making

Garland CW. World of practice: early intervention programs. In: Garner H, Orelove F, eds. Teamwork in Human Service Services: Models and Applications Across the Lifespan. Boston: Butterworth Heinemann, 1994:89–116.

disciplinary team evaluation of a high school adolescent with severe, multiple disabilities; and a medically oriented team evaluation of a child with feeding and swallowing concerns are provided as examples of team evaluations.

TEAM MEMBERS WHO COMMONLY WORK WITH OCCUPATIONAL THERAPISTS IN PEDIATRICS

Parents or Caregivers and Child

Most important, the child's **parents or caregivers** must be viewed as integral members of the team of individuals working together for the benefit of the child. When children are old enough, it is important to include them as well. Aside from their legal rights to participate in their child's evaluation process and intervention planning, caregivers know their child best and have the greatest stake in their child's well-being and future. They bring a wealth of information about their child to the evaluation process and help guide the intervention planning process by sharing their priorities and their child's strengths and challenges. The degree to which parents are involved depends on various factors, including the practice setting, parent preference, the age of the child, and the type and severity of disability.

General and Special Education Teachers and Teacher's Assistants

Educators are an integral part of the lives of all children as they move through the preschool and school years. **Special education teachers** have many roles with children who have been identified as requiring specialized instruction. First, they are involved in the student evaluation process and in the development of individual education programs (IEPs). Special educators are specifically trained in the administration of achievement tests and the evaluation of other behaviors important for learning and success at school. Second, they often provide direct instruction and implement portions of the IEP. They are particularly skilled in addressing cognitive development and learning styles and in instructional methods and development of curriculum for individual students with learning differences. For some students, this may mean modifying existing curriculum to assist students with academic skills such as reading and writing; for others, it may mean assisting in the development of an individualized curriculum that includes goals and objectives to promote life skills. Many special educators have expertise in the use of computer educational software and hardware. For children with severe disabilities, they are often involved in developing educational programs that consist largely of activities that address basic life skills, including activities of daily living, communication skills, and community and vocational skills. Third, special educators often take on many leadership roles, including liaison between the school and the parents; supervisor, teacher, and supporter of general education teachers and teacher's aides; and student case manager.

Teacher's assistants, sometimes referred to as paraprofessionals or teacher's aides, have the important role of assisting children with their daily functioning in the classroom. They may support children during academic subjects, assist in implementing behavioral support programs, and assist with self-care activities such as feeding and toileting. These individuals often spend more direct one-on-one time with children with special needs than any other team member and may communicate frequently with parents. Often, teacher's aides are given the responsibility of implementing many aspects of a child's education program with direction and support from the other team members, including the classroom teacher and related service providers such as occupational therapists.

Most children who require special education receive specialized instruction within the context of regular classroom activities and environments. Therefore, **general education teachers** are important team members for all of their students who receive special education. Throughout the evaluation and program planning process, the child's classroom teacher brings valuable ecologic information about the child's curriculum, classroom environment, and daily activities and about his or her own teaching style. General education teachers have a good understanding of the child's classroom behavior and needs and learning style. Often, general education teachers are responsible for implementing portions of a child's IEP and for monitoring the effectiveness of the program.

Occupational therapists often assist educators (special and general education teachers and aides) in designing education programs and in modifying school environments, curriculum, and classroom activities to maximize a child's ability to learn, function, and participate fully. With many children with special needs being fully included in regular education classes, it is more important than ever for occupational therapists to assist and support teachers in their efforts to provide quality programs and educational experiences for all children.

Physical Therapists

Physical therapists work with occupational therapists in medical, educational, and early-intervention environments. Pediatric physical therapy focuses on children's motor development or functional movement, which includes their ability to move and explore their environments, the development of fine and gross motor skills, and the performance of functional and play skills that are affected by movement disorders (Tatarka et al., 2000). The role of physical therapists and occupational therapists overlap a great deal with respect to the evaluation of motor skills and functional skills that are affected by movement disorders. Occupational therapists also work closely with physical therapists when evaluating the positioning needs of children, such as the need for wheelchairs or other specialized devices such as prone standers. For children with more severe disabilities and those in acute care and rehabilitation programs, physical therapists have a role in pain management and may work with occupational therapists in the prevention and management of joint contractures. In school settings, physical therapists may address a child's gross motor skills and assist with physical education or adapted physical education needs. Physical therapists have an important role in addressing children's safety and independence with mobility in school environments, including the proper use of mobility devices such as wheelchairs and walkers.

Speech-Language Pathologists

Speech-language pathologists, sometimes referred to as communication specialists or speech therapists, are responsible for evaluating and treating the communication abilities of children. They are trained at the Master's level to apply theories, principles, and procedures related to the development and disorders of language and speech for the purposes of assessment and treatment (American Speech-Language-Hearing Association, 2001). Because there is a close anatomical and functional relationship between the structures used for speaking and those used for eating and swallowing, they also assist with the management of feeding problems and dysphagia. Speech therapists' and occupational therapists' roles overlap in the area of feeding, particularly with respect to addressing the oral-motor control and swallowing abilities of children.

Because language is a cognitive skill, speech pathologists also have a role in addressing cognitive deficits, particularly those related to the promotion of functional language and communication. Addressing a child's communication abilities may require the use of assistive technology and augmentative communication devices. Therefore, occupational therapists often work closely with speech therapists in the evaluation and selection of appropriate communication devices, particularly for children with sensory motor deficits.

Certified Occupational Therapy Assistants

The role of certified occupational therapy assistants (COTAs) is described in a document by the American Occupational Therapy Association (1993) as being responsible for providing occupational therapy services to assigned clients under the supervision of registered occupational therapists. They may work closely with you in various settings. In terms of evaluation, COTAs may assist in the data collection process of an evaluation under the supervision of registered occupational therapists, including the administration of standardized tests, provided that an acceptable level of competency has been demonstrated. It is important to include COTAs in the evaluation and intervention planning process for children who they will be working with or with whom they have worked in the past.

Nurses

In school settings, **nurses** have an important role in the management of children who are medically fragile and have routine medical needs, such as the dispensing of medication, skin care, and first aid needs; feeding procedures such as tube feeding; and elimination needs such as catheterization. They may work with occupational therapists to help students develop independence with routine procedures or to train others, such as teachers and teacher's assistants, to safely administer some of these procedures. School nurses often speak frequently with parents and can update the team on medical concerns or needs to be considered during the development and implementation of a child's IEP.

Nurses are often part of early-intervention teams (Collins, 1995; Magyary et al., 2000). They may serve a variety of roles, such as case manager; assisting in the diagnosis of health and developmental problems of children and their families; helping families access early-intervention services; and assisting in the development and implementation of individual family service plans. Nurses make up the largest segment of the health care workforce. In acute, neonatal, and rehabilitation settings, they often take on the primary caregiving role and the case manager role. In hospital settings, it is important that you, as the occupational therapist, consult the nursing staff before entering a child's room to conduct evaluation procedures. Nurses and nursing assistants provide valuable information regarding the child's medical status and any precautions that need to be implemented during your evaluation. A child's medical/health status is always top priority; therefore, your evaluation (and intervention services) may need to be postponed at times owing to scheduling of medical procedures or because the child is not feeling well enough.

In hospital settings, the roles of nurses and occupational therapists often overlap with respect to the management of self-help skills such as bathing, dressing, toileting, functional mobility, and feeding.

Psychologists

In school, preschool, and medical settings, the roles of **psychologists** are to address a child's intellectual and adaptive abilities and psychosocial and emotional functioning (Hay and Breiger, 2000). They often provide services for evaluating and supporting a child's educational programming needs or mental health needs, and they may play a key role in diagnosing mental health conditions such as attention-deficit hyperactivity disorder and learning disorders. Psychologists are social scientists with training usually at the doctorate level, with expertise in the areas of human behavior, cognition, and psychological health. Therefore, as a member of a team working with children with disabilities, they typically evaluate the psychosocial, emotional, and behavioral abilities and needs of children as well as areas of cognitive functioning and learning styles. Psychologists may also provide direct services such as assisting with the design, implementation, and evaluation of behavioral support plans. School psychologists may consult with regular and special education teachers, assist in the development of IEPs, and provide direct counseling services for children and their families.

Physicians

A child's primary **physician** is usually a pediatrician or a family practitioner. Often, it is the primary physician who first identifies that a child may be at risk for developing problems or has a developmental or other concern. Therefore, physicians have an important role in referring appropriate children for evaluations and other early-intervention services.

In school settings, physicians (pediatricians, pediatric neurologists, and psychiatrists) have few roles, and they rarely communicate with school personnel on a regular basis. It is, however, important for physicians to be involved when children are medically fragile, when the school team requires information on the effects of medications, or when other medical conditions affect a child's ability to participate in school activities. The school nurse or a parent may function as a liaison between a child's physician and the rest of the school team. In addition, in the United States, some states require a physician's referral for the provision of related services in schools, such as physical and occupational therapy.

In medical settings, the physician is often viewed as the leader of the team. He or she writes the referrals for other team members and manages the child's medical needs. Children with disabilities often have complex medical needs; therefore, many physicians, such as those specializing in orthopedics, psychiatry, or neurology, may consult with the team on a regular basis.

Social Workers

Social workers help children and their families participate in their social environments. Depending on the needs of a family, social workers may be involved in assisting the child and family to secure necessary mental health or other resources, respite care, and financial support and services, and they may provide ongoing emotional support. According to Cook (2000), the role of social work with children is to assess, support, and empower the child's family so that they gain the resources, knowledge, and skills to optimize their child's growth and development. More specifically, they evaluate the needs of the family, and they may provide counseling services in various school and medical settings. Often they take the role of case manager to ensure that children and their families receive comprehensive and coordinated services.

Other Team Members

Many professionals and individuals in addition to those mentioned previously may be involved as members of a child's team. For example, dentists, nutritionists, adapted physical education and recreation specialists, mental health counselors, members of clergy, family advocates, and friends are just a few of the others who may have important roles for any given child and family. Team composition depends on the desires, resources, and needs of each individual child and family. It is also important to note that some members may be involved to a lesser extent than others, again depending on the needs of the child and family.

TYPES OF TEAMS

All types of teams serving children and their families are similar in that membership consists of the child, important individuals in the child's life, and professionals from a variety of different disciplines. However, types of teams often differ from one another with respect to the extent and type of collaboration among the team members, the degree to which they share roles, and their organizational structures and operational procedures. Table 6-1 provides a comparison of multidisciplinary, interdisciplinary, and transdisciplinary teams, which are the most common types of team models used for providing educational and health care services.

Multidisciplinary Teams

In a **multidisciplinary team**, the team members from various disciplines work with the same child but on an individual basis. Members may meet regularly, such as once a week, once a month, or on an as-needed basis, to discuss the child. On some multidisciplinary teams, members may just meet or talk informally. However, it is important that team members share information with one another to ensure that the child is receiving a comprehensive program, to share progress and other information, and to avoid duplication of services. Multidisciplinary teams work best in situations in which the child's needs are distinct from one another and when discipline-specific roles are well established. It is important that the contributions of each member are valued and that members perceive one another as having equal importance or status (Case-Smith, 2001).

TABLE 6-1 | COMPARISON OF MULTIDISCIPLINARY, INTERDISCIPLINARY, AND TRANSDISCIPLINARY TEAM MODELS

	Multidisciplinary	Interdisciplinary	Transdisciplinary
Evaluation procedures	Each discipline plans and does his or her evaluation separately	Team members collaborate to develop the evaluation plan; each discipline may conduct his or her own part of the evaluation separately or with other team members	Team members collaborate to develop the evaluation plan; team conducts the evaluation together, usually with one or two members working directly with the child while others observe
Program planning	Team meets to share findings; members develop separate plans for their disciplines	Team meets to share and synthesize findings; team collaborates to develop an intervention plan, which often includes discipline-specific interventions	Team meets to share findings; team collaborates to develop an intervention plan that is implemented by one or two individuals; all primary service provider(s) implements the plan
Communication	Informal; infrequent	Regular meetings; frequent informal contact	Frequent meetings; continuous contact among members with the direct service provider(s) for support, supervision, sharing of knowledge and skills, and assistance with program changes as needed
Program implementation	Team members implement the part of the program that reflects their area of expertise	Team members implement the part of the program that reflects their area of expertise; may provide co-treatment sessions and incorporate goals from other disciplines	A primary service provider is assigned to implement the program with the child and family, with ongoing support from the team members

As a member of a multidisciplinary team, you as the occupational therapist may need to communicate with other team members before your evaluation to ensure that you do not repeat evaluations of developmental areas unnecessarily. For example, if the speech pathologist has just conducted a thorough evaluation of oral-motor skills and swallowing, it may not be necessary for you to thoroughly assess these areas as a part of your feeding evaluation. Once the roles of team members are well established, then the need for this initial checking may be diminished. Under this team model, occupational therapists function relatively independently during the evaluation process, and the evaluation techniques provided in the earlier chapters of this book are applicable. In addition, you, as the occupational therapist, would be responsible for developing a separate occupational therapy plan when intervention services are recommended.

After all members of a multidisciplinary team have completed their evaluations, they commonly schedule a meeting to share their findings and intervention plans and strategies. The main purpose of these meetings is to allow for some coordination of services, including scheduling of services to maximize the efficiency of the services being offered by the team and to check that all the needs of the child and family are being addressed adequately. Ongoing communication often takes place in the form of documentation, which occurs regularly in the child's medical chart in hospital settings and via individual education plans in educational settings. It is important for team members to share with one another the child's progress in the areas they are working on and to ensure that the child is not receiving interventions that are counterproductive. Interventions from various professionals are most effective when they complement or reinforce one another, and this is particularly true for interventions that address behavioral difficulties.

Interdisciplinary Teams

Similar to multidisciplinary teams, **interdisciplinary teams** consist of professionals from various disciplines. However, an interdisciplinary team model has a formal structure for interaction and sharing of information among the team members and a higher degree of collaboration. For example, team members may conduct components of their evaluations and interventions with one another. Guralnick (2000) described interdisciplinary teams as having the ability to integrate and synthesize information from numerous disciplines through an interactive group decision-making process.

A typical interdisciplinary team evaluation begins with data gathering (medical record review, background information, medical history, etc.) by a team coordinator. Then, a team meeting is conducted to share and discuss the background information gathered and to plan the evaluation (see Figure 6-1). The third step consists of discipline-specific evaluations. In some cases, discipline-specific evaluations may be conducted jointly. For example, evaluations of motor performance may be conducted jointly by occupational and physical therapists. During this step, informal meetings and sharing of information among various disciplines may occur. The final step is a formal meeting to integrate and synthesize all of the information gathered by the team members. The team members, including the parents, collaborate and engage

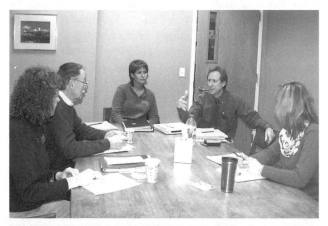

Figure 6–1. Example of an interdisciplinary team meeting consisting of a clinic coordinator, psychologist, speech pathologist, developmental pediatrician, and occupational therapist.

in group problem solving and decision making to identify the child's strengths, challenges, and needs; to develop intervention goals and plans; and to identify the need for further services and evaluations.

One of the main differences between a multidisciplinary team and an interdisciplinary team is that the members of an interdisciplinary team must reach consensus with respect to all of the recommendations made by the team. In contrast, multidisciplinary team members typically share their own recommendations with one another but do not necessarily work together to develop consensus. Another characteristic of interdisciplinary teams is that they can apply **integrated programming** techniques. Integrated programming occurs when a professional from one discipline incorporates the goals of another discipline into his or her interventions or when team members from two different disciplines work together (co-treatment sessions) with a child.

Transdisciplinary Teams

As with multidisciplinary and interdisciplinary teams, **transdisciplinary teams** recognize the need to include specialists or disciplines with expertise in several skill areas as well as the child (when old enough) and the parents. This team model is based on the assumption that services for families are most effective when the family is required to interact directly and regularly with only one or two key individuals. The most distinguishing characteristic of transdisciplinary teams is that only one or two individuals are primarily responsible for carrying out the child's intervention program. In educational settings, the key individual and direct service provider is most often an educator. In other settings, the direct service provider may be a developmental specialist or an occupational therapist. Transdisciplinary teams are often practiced in early-intervention and educational settings, particularly with children with more severe, multiple disabilities.

The prefix "trans" means "across," and it refers to the sharing of skills, responsibilities, and knowledge among team members. A key feature of the transdisciplinary team model is **role release**: the commitment of professionals to teaching, learning, and providing direct services that may not be traditionally within their discipline-specific roles. It does not, however, imply a transfer of ultimate professional responsibilities for an individual in his or her area of expertise or a dilution of high-quality services. Instead, the transdisciplinary team model stresses an integration of expertise that facilitates the development of coordinated, comprehensive programs for children. For team members other than the direct service provider, indirect methods of service delivery, including consultation, supervision, and monitoring, and ongoing support are applied.

Similar to interdisciplinary teams, transdisciplinary teams are structured in a way that facilitates the use of integrated programs but at a higher level than was described in the context of an interdisciplinary team. Integrated programs are developed collaboratively by transdisciplinary team members and comprise carefully selected program activities or functional skills that address more than one programming goal (Campbell, 1987). For example, an activity of watering plants in a classroom or hospital room might be designed by team members in such a way that the activity simultaneously addresses functional mobility, upper-extremity strength and coordination, ability to follow directions, and communication skills. This activity could be easily carried out by the child under the direction of or with the assistance of one direct service provider.

In terms of evaluation, a transdisciplinary team model conducts what has been termed an **arena assessment**. An arena assessment begins like an interdisciplinary team assessment in that background information is gathered by one or two individuals and then is shared among team members. Then, the evaluation process is carefully planned collaboratively. What makes an arena assessment unique is that the "hands-on" portion of the evaluation is often carried out by only one or two key individuals. The remainder of the team members provide their expertise through consultation, and they gather the information they require through observation, viewing the child from their individual discipline-specific perspectives. Arena assessments are particularly helpful when evaluating a child's ability to perform functional skills that require a variety of underlying sensory, motor, communication, social-emotional, and cognitive skills. For example, evaluations of computer access and technology needs and of feeding skills can often be accomplished using an arena format.

The Transdisciplinary Play-based Assessment (Linder, 1993) is an evaluation tool designed specifically as a transdisciplinary arena assessment. The purpose of this assessment is to gather information about the child's developmental skills by observing the child during unstructured play activities. A system is used for parents and professionals to plan, observe, and analyze collaboratively the child's skills through play.

A word of caution about using arena assessments: the number of people present for the assessment may be overwhelming for the child and family. Although typically only one or two individuals work directly with the clients, three to five others may be observing. It is important to be sensitive to the needs of the child and family and to ask them about their comfort level with all the proposed evaluation activities during the planning phase. This initial checking will help minimize the potential for encountering uncomfortable situations and will help prepare the family for the arena assessment.

EXAMPLE OF AN INTERDISCIPLINARY EVALUATION IN AN EARLY-INTERVENTION SETTING

Background Information and Evaluation Planning

System considerations include legislation supporting early-intervention services. Children from birth to 3 years of age are typically provided with community-based, family-centered services as defined under the IDEA, Part C (1997). This case begins with a referral that was received by an early-intervention community agency to evaluate and provide services to a child 8 months of age with Down's syndrome. The team coordinator (a developmental specialist with a degree in developmental psychology) reviewed the medical information and interviewed the mother and the referring physician (the child's pediatrician) by telephone. The team (consisting of the coordinator, a speech therapist, a physical therapist, an occupational therapist, and a nutritionist) then met to share relevant background and medical information and to plan the evaluation.

Early-intervention teams often use developmental screening and evaluation tools that are multifaceted or divided into specific sections or developmental areas. These tools may be administered by one team member who is skilled in evaluating all areas, or the administration process can be divided up so that different team members administer the portions of the test that reflect their areas of expertise.

Conducting the Evaluation

The team decided on the following evaluation activities, which were conducted during a 1-hour home visit:

1. Administration of the Hawaii Early Learning Profile (Furuno et al., 1984). The coordinator completed the personal/social, self-help, cognition, and communication domains, and the occupational therapist and physical therapist together completed the fine motor and gross motor test items, along with clinical observations of movement, oral-motor control, and postural control factors. Although the Hawaii Early Learning Profile (Furuno et. al., 1984) was used in this case, other developmental screening and evaluation tools are available to evaluate multiple domains of development and are useful for interdisciplinary, early-intervention teams (see Table 4-4).
2. The occupational therapist interviewed the parents regarding their priorities, occupations, and needs.
3. The coordinator, occupational therapist, and physical therapist observed the child during some unstructured, free play time with a variety of play materials and toys and during interactions with her parents.

In addition to the home visit, the team's nutritionist scheduled a separate evaluation session with the mother to review nutritional concerns and to collect assessment data specifically on intake.

Concluding the Evaluation

After the evaluation activities were finished, each discipline completed a written summary of their impressions and clinical observations and prepared for an interdisciplinary team meeting. During this meeting, the team members, including the parents, further synthesized the evaluation data and collaborated to identify the child's strengths, challenges, and programming needs. During this meeting, the intervention planning phase began by creating an initial draft of the individual family service plan. After this meeting, the coordinator compiled and integrated evaluation data from all of the team members involved and developed one comprehensive team evaluation report. This report provided the formal documentation of the team's evaluation and was signed by all team members who participated in the evaluation process (see Fig. 6-2).

EXAMPLE OF A TRANSDISCIPLINARY EVALUATION OF A HIGH SCHOOL CHILD WITH SEVERE DISABILITIES

Relevant Background Information and Evaluation Planning Activities

System considerations for this evaluation include legislation that supports education and vocational services for adolescents, including Vocational Rehabilitation Services and the IDEA, Part B (1997). At the time of the evaluation, the student, Mandy, was 16 years of age and was beginning the 11th grade. She was spending approximately half of her school day in a contained, special education classroom/program and half of her day in regular education classrooms, with the assistance of a

---

Interdisciplinary Developmental Evaluation
Northeast Community Early Intervention Services
26 Crane Dr. Dover, NH 03824
(603) 888-1111

Child's Name: *Johnny D.*
Date of Birth: *09/05/01*
Date of Evaluation: *April 10, 2002*
Parents' Names, Address, Telephone Number:

Referring Physician: *Dr P. Brooks, pediatrician*
Diagnosis: *Down's syndrome*
Team members Involved in the Evaluation: *Mr & Mrs D (child's parents), Johnny (child), Jane (occupational therapist), Mark (physical therapist), Heather (speech therapist), Joanne (developmental specialist; coordinator)*

Summary of Evaluation Activities

- Review of relevant medical records, telephone interview with Dr Brooks, referring physician
- Home visit to conduct parent interviews, administer the Hawaii Learning Profile (HELP) completed by occupational therapist, physical therapist, and developmental specialist; observe social play behaviors, sensory motor skills, and feeding skills
- Team meeting to share and synthesize evaluation data

Relevant Background Information:

Johnny is an 8-month-old infant with global developmental delays. He resides with his parents and 6-year-old brother Max. His mother had a healthy full term pregnancy with Johnny, and there were no complications with his delivery. Johnny was 6 pounds at birth, and his condition of Down's syndrome was recognized immediately owing to low muscle tone (hypotonia) and typical facial features. Later, genetic testing confirmed trisomy 21. Johnny experienced some difficulty with nursing early on but was discharged from the hospital after 3 days. Aside from frequent upper respiratory tract and ear infections, Johnny's medical health has been unremarkable. His height and weight are between the 25th and 50th percentiles for children with Down's syndrome. He has not yet had formal hearing and vision testing, although he has been monitored at well-baby visits, and no concerns have been reported.

Johnny's family recently moved to Dover from Maine. Johnny received early intervention services from 4–6 months of age once a week through an early intervention agency in Maine. The parents' current priorities are to obtain services to help Johnny continue to develop his motor, language, play, and feeding skills. Mom works part-time as a receptionist, Dad is a mechanic, and their older son is in first grade. Johnny goes to a family day center while mom is at work, and mom reported that she has been pleased with his care there.

Figure 6–2. Example of an early-intervention interdisciplinary developmental evaluation. *(continued)*

Figure 6–2. *(Continued)*

Assessment Results Based on the HELP Strands, Interview, and Observations

Sensory Regulation and Organization: Johnny is easily quieted when upset, by holding him or nursing, and he seems to need a great deal of physical contact. He rarely self-calms, and attempts at using a pacifier have been unsuccessful. He does not like frolic play. He has extended periods of 3–4 hours when he is alert, and he shows an active interest in people and objects in his environment.

Cognition: Johnny is alert and aware of his surroundings when awake and ready to play. Cognitive skills range from the 3- to 4-month level. Johnny can hold and shake a rattle. He seems interested in exploring simple cause-effect toys, and he uses his hands and mouth to explore. He will bang objects. He will look toward sounds and voices and visually track objects. He does not look for hidden objects, but will react when a desired object is removed from view. He reaches for objects purposely that are within his reach, but he rarely attempts to reach objects that are out of his reach. Johnny is interested in looking at his hands and will repeat a simple newly learned activity like banging an object. He will not imitate simple gestures.

Language: Language/communication skills range from the 2- to 4-month level. Johnny inconsistently will watch those who are speaking to him. He does not look or vocalize to his name, wave bye-bye, or lift his arms when he wants to be held. He does not yet babble, but his cries vary in pitch and volume, and he vocalizes attitudes such as squealing and cooing.

Gross Motor Skills: Johnny exhibits low muscle tone throughout his body, with skills ranging from the 3- to 4-month old level. In prone, he can lift his head and chest and weight bear on his forearms. In supine, he kicks reciprocally, brings his hands to midline, and can maintain his head in midline. He cannot yet bring his feet to his mouth or lift his head in supine. He can sit with minimal support, can hold his head up without bobbing, and is beginning to move his head in supported sitting. He bears little weight on his legs when placed in supported standing. Johnny can roll from prone to supine, but not supine to prone. Evidence of the Moro reflex and asymmetrical tonic neck reflex were present. He demonstrated head righting reactions but not body righting reactions, or protective extension reactions. Held in ventral suspension, he could lift his head in line with the body, and in a pull to sit from supine, he demonstrated complete head lag.

Fine Motor Skills: Johnny visually tracks objects, although he cannot yet follow without head movement. He reaches for objects and will use an ulnar palmar grasp to hold objects. He cannot yet release objects or hold onto tiny objects, and he demonstrates fine motor skills at the 3- to 4-month level. His grasp reflex is inhibited, and his hands are open more than 50% of the time. He can clasp his hands together.

Social-emotional: Johnny does not display separation anxiety, and his parents describe him as an easy baby. He will establish eye contact and draw attention to himself by crying when in distress. He is

Figure 6–2. *(Continued)*

beginning to explore himself, including looking at and mouthing his hands, and seems interested in adult faces. He will smile and squeal to display happiness or excitement, with skills ranging from the 5- to 6-month level.

Self-help Skills: Johnny is nursing full-time, with the exception of feedings at day care, where he will drink breast milk from a bottle. Attempts have been made to introduce baby foods, but Johnny is not interested. Mom is comfortable to continue with nursing, but would like to continue trying baby foods. An attempt to feed Johnny baby food fruit and cereal was unsuccessful, as Johnny began to scream. Oral-motor evaluation indicated that his tongue movements are sluggish, he has excessive drooling, and he continues to demonstrate a rooting reflex. Sucking, swallowing, and breathing are adequately coordinated. He cannot yet hold his bottle. Generally, Johnny naps for 3 hours in the morning, and 3–4 hours in the afternoon. He wakes 1–2 times during the night wanting to nurse, and he tends to go back to sleep quite easily.

Summary:

Johnny is a healthy infant who seems well attached to his parents and who is ready to explore and learn from his environment. His skills across developmental areas range from the 3- to 5-month level, approximately 3–4 months below his chronological age of 8 months. Like many children with Down's syndrome, he has relative strength in the area of social-emotional skills. He is eligible for early intervention supports, and his individual family services plan is in the process of being developed collaboratively with his parents. He lives in a wonderfully supportive family, and his parents report that they are managing his care without difficulty and becoming more connected in their new community.

Based on this evaluation, the early-intervention team has made the following general recommendation: weekly home visits by the developmental specialist, with monthly consultations with the occupational therapist, physical therapist, and speech therapist. In addition, a weekly play group run by an occupational therapist and assistants is available. It is felt that Johnny and his parents would benefit from this experience, which includes programming for Johnny and a parent support and education component. Johnny's programming will focus on the development of feeding skills, play skills, ability to communicate, and gross and fine motor skills. In addition, support will be provided to his family as needed to assist with community integration, such as consulting with his day care providers to assist them in providing a successful experience for Johnny, and with helping the family access community resources that would be of benefit to them.

Signatures of Team Members:

full-time teacher's assistant. Mandy has Rhett syndrome, with significant cognitive impairment, and motor deficits such that she depends on others to push her in her manual wheelchair (her main means of mobility), and she has little functional movement of the upper extremities. Mandy also has a poorly controlled seizure disorder. Because this child is older than 14 years, transition planning and programming is an essential part of her IEP.

Mandy's education team included her special education teacher; mother; teacher's assistant; occupational, speech, and physical therapists; and school nurse. The team met to plan her 3-year evaluation, which is mandated under the IDEA. The team was familiar with this child and had worked with her in the past; therefore, little review of past records was necessary. However, a careful review of past IEP goals and educational strategies was conducted so that team members had a good understanding of what she had been working on and of the effectiveness of teaching strategies that had been tried in the past. Mandy's mother was very helpful in sharing Mandy's medical concerns regarding the control of her seizures and her medication regimen and with expressing her needs, wants, and dreams for Mandy and her priorities for Mandy's educational program.

The transdisciplinary team agreed to use the following evaluation activities: a parent interview, which was conducted during the planning meeting; a structured ecological assessment tool called a curriculum wheel, which was completed by her mother and teachers; completion of a form called a current-next-eventual form completed by her parents; and observations of Mandy during three school activities (feeding during lunch, computer time, and adapted physical education). These evaluation activities were conducted in an arena format.

Description of Evaluation Tools and Activities

Transdisciplinary team evaluations of children with severe/profound or multiple disabilities are helpful because it is often difficult to separate the influence of sensory, motor, communication, psychosocial, and cognitive abilities on the performance of functional skills. Also, the performance of functional skills depends on contextual factors and task demands, in combination with the child's underlying abilities. Because the specific contribution of each of these skill areas to the performance of the task is sometimes difficult to sort out, having professionals from multiple disciplines viewing the child performing the same task from multiple viewpoints is very useful. Collaborative arena evaluations reduce the risk of duplication and redundancy during an evaluation and provide all team members with a common basis or experience from which to synthesize evaluation data for intervention planning.

The curriculum wheel is an ecologic evaluation and was helpful for prioritizing the areas that were most important to the child and family while considering contextual factors and only relevant, meaningful functional activities. Evaluation guidelines by Orelove and Sobsey (1991) provided a helpful framework for conducting this ecologic evaluation. They suggest starting the evaluation process by identifying the environments and subenvironments in which the child currently functions, organized by the following four domains: home and self-care activities, school and educational activities, community activities, and recreational and leisure activities. For example, under the domain of home and self-care activities, the environment would be the family home and the subenvironments might include specific rooms such as the bedroom and kitchen. At school, subenvironments might be the cafeteria, the gym, and specific classrooms. Then, within each subenvironment, the activities or tasks that the child is required to do, typically does, or would like to learn to do are identified. Finally, the specific skills that are required to perform the activities are identified. This process is similar to an activity analysis in that the specific component skills necessary to complete certain functional skills are identified. The end product of this type of ecology inventory resembles a map, which details the activities that need to be addressed in a program, where they need to be addressed, and what areas or underlying skills need to be targeted (see the curriculum wheel in Fig. 6-3). This evaluation tool also uses the top-down system described in Chapter 2, as the process begins by identifying the contexts and functional skills that the child is expected to do first and only then considers the task demands and specific components or child factors required to complete the skill.

The current-next-eventual form is a tool that is useful when evaluating children who have multiple disabilities, including severe and profound mental retardation. This tool provided an opportunity for Mandy's family members to address issues of quality of life and to fully explore and share their priorities and dreams for Mandy. The current-next-eventual form asks caregivers to write down on a form what their child currently can do and what their child is expected to do. Then they are asked to think about and write down what they would like their child to learn to do next (within the next 1–2 years) and what they would like their child to eventually be able to do (within the next 5–10 years). This exercise is useful for uncovering parent priorities and values, and it encourages parents to think a little bit into the future. The timelines used to determine the "next" and "eventual" can be individualized. Although looking into the future is always a difficult task, thinking about what is important for the child's future provides essential guidance for developing effective individual programs and provides a basis for developing and implementing transition plans.

Three separate education-related activities that were components of Mandy's program throughout her week at school were carefully selected as the basis of the arena assessment: feeding during lunch, computer time, and adapted physical education time. These specific activities were selected because they could be viewed in natural contexts; they would provide necessary information regarding sensory, motor, communication, cognitive, and social-emotional abilities; and they represented functional skills of value to Mandy and her family. The team member that was primarily responsible for establishing her programming goals and objectives around these activities carried out the

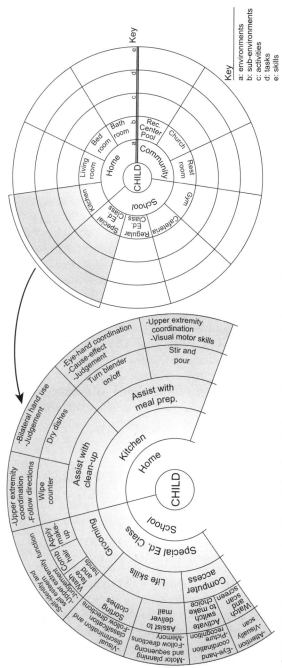

Figure 6–3. Curriculum wheel for a high school student with severe, multiple disabilities.

Key

a: environments
b: sub-environments
c: activities
d: tasks
e: skills

evaluation activity with Mandy while the other team members observed.

Concluding the Evaluation

The process of concluding the evaluation was similar to what was described in the early-intervention example. After the evaluation activities were completed, each discipline completed a written summary of their impressions and observations and prepared for a team meeting. During the team meeting, the team members, including parents, further synthesized the evaluation data and collaborated to identify the child's strengths, challenges, and programming needs. During this meeting, the intervention planning phase began by creating an initial draft of the IEP and a transition plan. Because of the need to develop a transition program, a representative from a community agency representing vocational rehabilitation services joined the team to share the types of programming options that would be available for Mandy after high school. After this meeting, the special education teacher, acting as case manager, compiled and integrated evaluation data from all of the team members involved and developed one comprehensive team evaluation report. The evaluation report provided the formal documentation of the team's evaluation and was signed off on by all team members who participated in the evaluation.

EXAMPLE OF AN INTERDISCIPLINARY TEAM EVALUATION OF A CHILD WITH DYSPHAGIA

Relevant Background Information and Evaluation Planning Activities

The child, 7-year-old Danny with cerebral palsy and spastic quadriplegia, was referred to a specialized feeding clinic for the evaluation of dysphagia and feeding difficulties. He was referred by his pediatrician after his school occupational therapist and mother expressed concerns about Danny's ability to swallow and his poor nutritional intake.

Feeding clinics are one of many specialty areas that often include occupational therapists as integral members of their evaluation teams. Setting and system considerations include medical insurance policies regarding reimbursement and the IDEA, Part B, as his school program would be implementing some of the recommendations made by this team. Some of the other pediatric specialty areas that also often include occupational therapists are clinics specializing in the evaluation of seating and positioning needs, neonatal care and follow-up, the evaluation of significant emotional and behavioral problems, and the evaluation and provision of assistive and augmentative communication devices and other high technological and computer equipment.

In this case, the team followed an interdisciplinary team model. The speech pathologist, acting as the case coordinator, collected and shared preliminary information with the other team members and scheduled the evaluation during a 2-hour block of time at the hospital's clinic. The team members included the parents, the coordinator/speech pathologist, the clinic occupational therapist (the school occupational therapist came to observe), a nutritionist, and a radiologist and a radiology technician. The morning of the evaluation, the team met briefly to finalize the evaluation activities, which included the following: discipline-specific evaluations by the nutritionist and the occupational therapist and videofluoroscopy conducted by the speech therapist, occupational therapist, radiologist, and technician.

Concluding the Evaluation

After the evaluation activities, the team coordinator and nutritionist met with the child and his parents and school occupational therapist to share immediate concerns and recommendations. A full report followed a couple of weeks later with the results of the team evaluation and more specific recommendations (see Fig. 6-4).

Child: *Danny*   **Date of Birth:** *June 1, 1995*   **Age:** *7 years*

Parents: **Address:**

Referring Physician:

Date of Evaluation: *July 12, 2002*

Reason for Referral: Danny has cerebral palsy and spastic quadriplegia and was referred for the evaluation of dysphagia and feeding difficulties. His school occupational therapist and mother expressed concerns about Danny's ability to swallow and his poor nutritional intake for obtaining desired weight gain and growth.

Team Members Present: Dr Brown, radiologist; radiology technician; C. Smith, MA CCC, speech-language pathologist and team coordinator; C. Jons, OTR, clinic occupational therapist; Patricia (child's mother), P. Anderson, MSOTR, school occupational therapist; J. Caron, nutritionist

Methods of Evaluation: Parent interview; discipline-specific evaluations by the nutritionist and occupational therapist; videofluoroscopy conducted by the speech therapist, occupational therapist, radiologist, and radiology technician, including the ability to swallow thin liquid, puree, crunchy quick-to-dissolve, honey consistency, and nectar consistency

Oral-Motor Control and Self-feeding: Danny is positioned in his power wheelchair for feeding, which includes lateral head supports, a lower-extremity abductor pad, and a chest strap to assist with his stability and to help him maintain an upright and symmetrical sitting posture. He can use both hands together to lift a sport-type drinking bottle, drink with a straw on his own, and bring his right hand to his mouth to finger feed. He has poorly controlled release of food items into his mouth and tends to use his lips to assist food to enter the mouth. He can hold an adapted spoon, which is angled and has a built-up handle, with his right hand. Pureed foods such as apple sauce are typically given in his lipped bowl with suction cups, and, with minimal physical assist to his right forearm, he can scoop food and spoon feed. He requires occasional verbal cues to sit up straight and reminders to flex his head slightly forward when swallowing. Danny has restricted, and poorly controlled oral-motor movements that affect feeding and speech. His tongue movements in particular are restricted by a tight frenulum, which is placed slightly more forward than what is typical.

Swallowing: The oral initiation phase is characterized by tongue movements in front to back action, to propel the food to the back of the tongue for swallowing. As the food or sips reach the back of the tongue, the soft palate lowers to create a seal. Danny both accepts food and will place food in his mouth. For all food consistencies he has a humped rather than bowled tongue configuration. Liquids spilled throughout his mouth and inside his cheeks and seeped under his tongue. He experienced difficulty with chewing, and tended to use weak up and down movements and no rotary chewing motions. He used his tongue and

Figure 6–4. Dysphagia team evaluation.

Figure 6–4. (Continued)

jaw movements to mash foods against the roof of his mouth and also used head movements to move food to the back of his molars.

The oral initiation phase is normally characterized by front-to-back tongue movements to propel food to the back of the tongue to initiate the swallow. The feeling of bolus of food against the back of the tongue, the soft palate, sends sensory information to various parts of the brain and triggers a series of contractions that begin the pharyngeal phase of the swallow. Danny is largely reliant on neck hyperextension to move the bolus to the back of the tongue. He cannot elevate his tongue effectively to initiate the swallow. Therefore, his swallow reflex is delayed.

The pharyngeal phase is characterized by closing of the epiglottis to prevent food from entering the trachea. The upper esophageal sphincter relaxes. The base of the tongue, soft palate, and walls at the back of the throat push the food into the pharynx and seal the passage into the nasal cavity. Peristaltic action pushes the food into the esophagus. Danny's reliance on neck hyperextension caused food and drink to spill prematurely into the pharynx. The swallow was initiated at the level of the pyriform sinuses for puree, crunchy/solid, and thickened drinks. For thin liquids, the swallow was initiated later, often once liquid had penetrated behind the epiglottis, and aspiration was noted with thin liquids on one occasion. For the nectar consistency, penetration occurred inconsistently and did not occur for the honey-thick consistency drink. Pureed food particles stayed in the pyriform sinuses and valleculae after the swallow, creating a further risk for aspiration. When this solid food was alternated with honey consistency drink, the food particles were effectively cleared from these cavities.

The esophageal phase is characterized by the transport of the bolus through the esophageal sphincter into the stomach. Danny's upper esophageal sphincter relaxed once the swallow reflex was triggered, allowing food and drink into the esophagus, and food and drink appeared to move smoothly through the upper esophagus.

Nutrition Evaluation: Data were collected by parent interview, measures of height and weight, and a 3-day food record. Danny's height/length was at the 10th percentile, and his weight was at the 5th percentile, compared with other children his age with cerebral palsy. His weight, based on his height, was at the 3rd percentile. Danny's diet consisted of fruit juices and milk (8 oz, five times per day) and Pediasure supplement (10 oz, once per day), three meals per day and two snacks, consisting mostly of pureed and soft foods such as yogurt, apple sauce, mashed fruit, vegetables, pasta, and rice. He could manage graham crackers and tiny bits of meat. Based on the 3-day food intake, his energy intake of 15 calories per centimeter of length was low, and growth parameters indicated that he was slightly underweight. His family was concerned about his lack of progress with his ability to manage solid foods and with his frequent coughing with thin liquids. Behaviorally, Danny was reported to enjoy eating for the most part, although he often got bored or tired before completing his meals. The length of time for completing a meal with assistance was approximately 45 minutes.

(continued)

Figure 6–4. (Continued)

Summary and Impressions:

Findings from this evaluation indicate that Danny has significant oral-motor dysfunction and mild-to-moderate pharyngeal phase dysphagia. His dysphagia seems to be the result of his neuromotor disorder and limited tongue mobility caused by the tight frenulum. Danny cannot bowl his tongue or lift his tongue adequately to initiate the swallow. He relies mostly on neck hyperextension, which effectively uses gravitational forces to propel the bolus and initiate the swallow reflex. This creates premature spilling of food into the pharynx and places him at high risk for aspiration with thin liquids and nectar consistency drinks. He could manage honey consistency drinks without significant difficulty. The pharyngeal phase also demonstrated reduced peristalsis, which results in residue being left in the pharynx. This residue was effectively cleared away by alternating solid food with sips of honey consistency drinks. Danny requires minimal to moderate assistance overall for self-feeding because of limited upper-extremity function and oral-motor control. He is motivated to participate in self-feeding as much as he is able. It takes him excessive amounts of time to complete a meal, and he uses some adapted equipment to promote self-feeding. His caloric intake is slightly lower than it should be given his activity level and height, and his growth needs to be monitored on a regular basis.

Recommendations: To minimize the risk of aspiration, Danny's drinks should be thickened to a honey-thick (shake) consistency. For example, juices can be thickened with blended fruits, baby foods, yogurt or Thick-it. Consultation with an ear-nose-throat specialist is recommended for further evaluation and possible surgical treatment of the attachment of his frenulum. Continue with his oral-motor program, with emphasis on developing his ability to bowl and move his tongue, improving chewing abilities and grading of jaw movements, and coordinating lip closure. His diet should be regularly monitored, with ongoing support from the nutritionist. It is recommended that his diet consist of mainly pureed foods, honey-thick liquids, foods that easily form a bolus, and quick-to-dissolve crunchy foods. Mixed consistency foods (such as soups) and thin liquids should be avoided. During meals, solid foods should be alternated with drinks. Continue programming to address and monitor his positioning needs and to promote his self-feeding abilities.

Further questions regarding the information in this report can be directed to C. Smith, MA CCC, speech-language pathologist and team coordinator at 112-112-1122.

Signatures of Team Members:

SUMMARY

This chapter provided an introduction of the roles of professionals from various disciplines who typically work closely with occupational therapists. It is important to recognize the child's parents or caregivers as full team members, as well as the child when old enough, throughout the planning, implementation, and sharing of evaluations. A clear understanding of the roles of the professionals on the teams you are on will help you define your responsibilities and will facilitate the selection and coordination of evaluation activities. Three types of team models—multidisciplinary, interdisciplinary, and transdisciplinary—were discussed, along with some examples of team evaluations. Because children with disabilities are complex, it is helpful for professionals from various disciplines to work together throughout the evaluation process to formulate the most accurate and comprehensive understanding of a child's disability, strengths, challenges, and programming needs. Finally, it is important that team members are aware of and attend to their team process every now and again. Like all good things in life, it takes work and nurturance for teams to function well. Therefore, taking the time to foster healthy team dynamics, to understand one another, and to revisit the specific philosophy and goals guiding the work of your team will aid in promoting a cohesive, pleasant, and efficient working atmosphere.

References

American Occupational therapy Association (1993). Occupational therapy roles. *American Journal of Occupational Therapy,* 47, 1087–1099.

American Speech-Language-Hearing Association (ASHA, 2001). Scope of practice in speech-language pathology, www.asha.org.

Case-Smith, J. (2001). Teaming. In J. Case-Smith (Ed.), *Occupational therapy for children* (4th ed., pp. 21–38), St. Louis, MO: Mosby, Inc.

Campbell, P.H. (1987). The integrated programming team: An approach for coordinating professionals of various disciplines in programs for students with severe and multiple handicaps. *Journal for the Association of Persons with Severe Handicaps,* 12(2), 107–116.

Collins, R.M. (1995). Nurses in early intervention. *Pediatric Nursing,* 21(6), 529–531.

Cook, D. (2000). The role of social work with families that have young children with developmental disabilities. In M. Guranl-nick (Ed.) *Interdisciplinary clinical assessment of young children with developmental disabilities* (p. 201–218). Baltimore, MD: P.H. Brookes Publishing Co., Inc.

Furuno, S., O'Reilly, K.A., Hosaka, C.M., Inatsuka, T., Allman, T.A., & Zeisloft, B.(1984). *The Hawaii early learning profile.* Palo Alto, CA: Vort Corporation.

Garland. C.W. (1994). World of practice: Early intervention pro-grams. In H. Garner & F. Orelove (Eds.), *Teamwork in human service services: Models and applications across the lifespan* (pp. 89–116). Boston, MA: Butterworth Heinemann.

Guralnick, M. (2000). Interdisciplinary team assessment for young children: Purposes and processes. In M. Guranlnick (Ed.), *Interdisciplinary clinical assessment of young children with developmental disabilities* (pp. 3–18). Baltimore, MD: P.H. Brookes Publishing Co., Inc.

Hay, A., & Breiger, A. (2000). Psychological assessment and the interdisciplinary team . In M. Guralnick (Ed.), *Interdiscipli-nary clinical assessment of young children with developmental disabilities* (pp. 183–199), Baltimore, MD: P.H. Brookes Pub-lishing Co., Inc.

Individuals with Disabilities Education Act (IDEA; 1997). Amendments of 1997 (PL.105-17). U.S.C. 1400.

Linder, T.W. (1993). Transdisciplinary play-based assessment: A functional approach to working with young children. Balti-more, MD: P.H. Brookes Co., Inc.

Magyary, D., Brant, P., & Kieckhefer, G. (2000). The nursing role in the interdisciplinary assessment team. In M. Guranlnick (Ed.), *Interdisciplinary clinical assessment of young children with developmental disabilities* (pp. 68–85). Baltimore, MD: P.H. Brookes Publishing Co., Inc.

McCormack, L., & Goldman, R. (1979). The transdisciplinary model: Implications for service delivery and personnel prepa-ration for the severely and profoundly handicapped. *AAESPH Review, 4*(2), 152–161.

Orelove, F., & Sobsey, D. (1991). *Educating children with multiple disabilities: A transdisciplinary approach* (2nd ed.). Baltimore, MD: P.H. Brookes Publishing Co., Inc.

Tatarka, M., Swanson, M., & Washington, K. (2000). The role of physical therapy in the interdisciplinary team process. In M. Guralnick (Ed.), Interdisciplinary clinical assessment of young children with developmental disabilities (pp. 130–151). Baltimore, MD: P.H. Brookes Publishing Co., Inc.

7

INTERVENTION PLANNING AND DOCUMENTATION

INTRODUCTION

The content covered in this chapter expands on the information presented in Chapter 2 on the final three steps of the evaluation process: synthesizing and summarizing evaluation data, intervention planning, and communicating evaluation results through verbal and written reports. Making sense of all the evaluation data you have collected and then planning an intervention are complex processes. Completion of these evaluation activities should ultimately result in a list of client strengths, challenges, and priorities and will provide you with the necessary direction for identifying intervention options and creating client-centered intervention programs. Important factors to consider as you engage in the **clinical reasoning** process for developing intervention plans are discussed in this chapter, with particular attention to the need for collaboration, making discharge projections, and applying the best available research. Practical skills for writing intervention goals and behavioral objectives are addressed in detail, and examples are included. The chapter concludes with information to assist you with communicating evaluation results through report writing and oral presentations such as those given during family and team meetings. Three sample occupational therapy initial evaluation reports are also provided.

DEVELOPING THE INTERVENTION PLAN

Collaborating With Others

Intervention planning, first and foremost, should be a **collaborative effort.** It is essential that you review evaluation results with the child's parents and with the child when he or she is old enough. Client involvement in the process helps ensure that child and family priorities are addressed and that practical considerations such as those related to scheduling are taken into consideration as the intervention program is developed. It is also important to share evaluation results and intervention planning ideas and recommendations with other individuals who are directly involved with the child's care and services, such as the child's teacher. **Parental consent** is, however, required before sharing evaluation information with others. Sharing your recommendations with other team members ensures that your proposed interventions are not overly redundant or contradictory with the services of others. In addition, it is effective if the intervention approaches and activities used by different disciplines complement or support those provided by others, when possible.

If you are working in educational settings, under the Individuals With Disabilities Education Act, Part B or Part C (1997), then your intervention program will be a part of a larger program. The development of individual education programs and individual family services plans are required by law to be collaborative processes.

In medical and community settings, **reimbursement for services** often needs to be discussed, and preapproval for intervention services may be necessary before finalizing your intervention program. Therefore, you may need to work with the family or reimbursement agency before implementing the proposed program.

Creating Long-Term Goals and Discharge Projections

Many factors contribute to your clinical reasoning as you develop intervention plans for children. It is suggested that you begin the process by identifying **long-term goals** or

functional outcomes that you, along with the child and family, believe are important and that can be realistically achieved as a result of occupational therapy intervention. Long-term goals are sometimes referred to as **discharge projections** in medical settings, and they represent the anticipated results or outcomes of your interventions. Discharge projections or long-term goals include what you hope your client will achieve, what you anticipate the child's functional status to be at the time therapy is discontinued, as well as how long you believe the child will require intervention.

Making predictions of the benefits or gains you anticipate a child will experience as a result of your intervention helps justify the medical or educational necessity for occupational therapy intervention services and often serves as essential documentation for insurance reimbursement. Making such predictions is not an easy task. To help with this process, consider the child's developmental history and response to interventions in the past. Also base your judgments on the research evidence provided in the literature and on your own clinical experience to determine the kinds of gains or outcomes that can be expected. It is also important to ask yourself what you would anticipate happening if occupational therapy services were not provided.

Applying Research Evidence

After your client's goals have been identified, you need to decide how you are going to go about helping your client accomplish his or her goals. Will your intervention be delivered directly? Will treatment be provided in a group or individually? Where will intervention services be conducted? Will your intervention be provided indirectly by a certified occupational therapy assistant, rehabilitation aide, or teacher? What specific therapy techniques and frames of reference will you use? The service delivery options available to you, specific child and family goals and preferences, and your skills all need to be considered as you develop intervention plans for individual clients.

One of the most important factors that you need to consider when developing intervention plans is the best available research evidence on the efficacy of the interventions you are considering. Research evidence is important for guiding your treatment considerations and ultimate decisions and will also assist you in making discharge projections. Using the research literature to guide clinical decision making has been termed **evidence-based practice**. This practice involves the integration of your clinical expertise and experiences with the application of the current, best research evidence in making decisions about the care of individual clients (Sackett et al., 1996). Evidence-based practice has been endorsed by our national professional organization (the American Occupational Therapy Association) as well as by most other educational and health care professional organizations. It is the ethical responsibility of occupational therapists to keep current on the research evidence, limitations, and scope of the interventions that are recommended and to share this information with clients. This information helps you identify the appropriate intervention options to consider for certain clients. In addition, sharing information gained from the synthesis of well-designed research studies helps the families you serve make informed decisions about whether to accept proposed intervention plans.

Once your long-term goals, approaches, intervention techniques, and service delivery methods have been determined, you need to determine the **scheduling** of your interventions. Scheduling involves determining the frequency and length of sessions and the location of the services. Family activities and schedules, type of client and intervention plan and goals, research evidence, reimbursement considerations, and your schedule all will impact scheduling decisions. Questions to aid you as you go through the process of synthesizing evaluation data for intervention planning are summarized in Box 7-1.

Writing Goals and Objectives

The purpose of writing goals and objectives is to help guide the intervention process, to communicate to others

BOX 7-1	QUESTIONS TO AID YOUR CLINICAL REASONING DURING EVALUATION PROCESS STEPS 10 TO 12

Step 10—Interpret, Synthesize, and Summarize Your Evaluation Data

What are the most important findings? What was the purpose of the evaluation, and have you answered the questions posed by the referral source? What objective data do you have to support your interpretations and impressions? What are the child's overall strengths and weaknesses? What are the child's and caregiver's priorities related to functional goals and abilities? What child factors, environmental/contextual factors, and activity demands are contributing to the child's successes and challenges in performing daily activities? What new information can you contribute about this child and his or her programming needs?

Step 11—Develop Recommendations and Intervention Planning

What are the parent and child priorities? What is feasible for them, and you, in consideration of your resources? What are other professionals addressing with the child? What is the research evidence supporting the interventions you are considering? What gains can you expect in response to intervention? What are your short- and long-term goals for this child?

Step 12—Document and Share Your Evaluation Results

Who is going to read your report? Have you addressed all of the referral questions? Is your report professionally written? Are your impressions clearly supported by objective evaluation data? How will you present the information concisely in a meeting?

what it is you are doing, and to provide a measure of intervention effectiveness or child progress. Goals are commonly divided into short term and long term. There is no "official standard" for determining the time frame that defines a long- or short-term goal. The time frame selected depends on various factors, including the child's condition, the anticipated rate of progress, and the setting or service delivery system.

Generally speaking, **long-term goals** reflect what you would like the child to be able to do at the time services are no longer needed, which relates to the anticipated results of your interventions. However, for children with chronic or progressive conditions, this might not always be applicable. In school settings, long-term goals are often established for a child's school year. In rehabilitation or other hospital settings, long-term goals might be written for a 3-month or a 3-week period only if that is the time frame you anticipate that the child will be hospitalized or require occupational therapy services.

It is important that long-term goals relate to a specific functional activity or occupation important to the child and that you define the time frame in which you expect the goal to be achieved. For example, a goal related to feeding performance might be: Within 3 months, Jack will be able to eat all three meals independently, with setup assistance only.

Short-term goals reflect the steps the child needs to accomplish or go through to meet his or her long-term goals. Short-term goals are often written as behavioral objectives so that they can be used as a means of measuring the child's progress toward the long-term goal. It is important that you select and write behavioral objectives carefully so that they are capable of helping you monitor, measure, and document the progress of the child. According to Zimmerman (1988), **behavioral objectives** include three main components:

1. **The Behavior:** The behavior is what you would like the child to be able to do.

2. **The Condition:** Conditions are factors that support the behavior, such as the type and level of assistance provided, use of adapted equipment, or any other environmental or situational factors. Conditions help define the range of the behavior and often define when, where, and in what context you will examine the behavior.

3. **The Criterion:** Criteria are set to provide a standard or measure for determining whether the child has achieved the desired behavior. Criteria used to measure performance are extremely variable and depend directly on the type of behaviors you wish to work on and measure. A common type of measurement criterion is the percentage of time the child does the desired behavior when requested. Qualitative descriptors may also be used as a type of criterion, and they

BOX 7-2	SAMPLE LONG-TERM GOALS FOR AN INPATIENT REHABILITATION SETTING

1. Within 2 months, Matthew will improve sitting and standing balance so that he can dress himself independently.

2. Within 2 months, Matthew will improve his ability to attend and concentrate so that he can work on homework activities for 20 min.

3. Within 2 months, when set up, Matthew will be able to feed himself, including the use of utensils independently.

define how the behavior needs to be demonstrated. For example, the criteria might be the level of assistance the child requires to perform the behavior.

Examples of long-term goals are provided in Boxes 7-2 to 7-4, and examples of behavioral objectives are provided in Boxes 7-5 and 7-6.

DOCUMENTATION AND SHARING OF INFORMATION

The final step in the evaluation process includes documentation of the evaluation and sharing of the information. Three **sample evaluation reports** documenting pediatric occupational therapy evaluations for different practice settings and ages of children are provided in Figures 7-1 to 7-3. Although

BOX 7-3	SAMPLE LONG-TERM GOALS FOR A SCHOOL SETTING

1. By the end of the school year, Carol will improve fine motor skills so that she can print her name legibly on top of her work papers.

2. By the end of the school year, Carol will improve her social skills so that she plays nicely with peers on the playground during recess.

3. By the end of the school year, Carol will be able to perform her morning routine of getting off of the bus, getting to her classroom, and putting her coat and belongings away independently.

BOX 7-4	SAMPLE LONG-TERM GOALS FOR AN OUTPATIENT CLINIC SETTING

1. Within 3 months, Johnny will decrease his tactile hypersensitivity so that at preschool he can play comfortably in the sand table and with art materials, including fingerpaint and Playdough.
2. Within 3 months, Johnny will improve motor planning abilities so that he can ride a tricycle independently.

there is some room for individual styles and preferences in the way reports are written, it is important that you follow specific formats for writing up evaluation reports required in your setting. At a minimum, the information included in the sample evaluation report outlined in Figure 7-4 should be included in all occupational therapy initial evaluation reports.

The most important section in an evaluation report is the **evaluation summary and impressions section**. This section is a synthesis of all of your evaluation data and is written in a concise way so that professionals who just want a quick summary of the evaluation can get the information they need in this section alone. The rest of the report should provide the detailed information that supports your summary and impressions.

It is recommended that when writing evaluation reports you choose language carefully so that all interested audi-

BOX 7-5	SAMPLE BEHAVIORAL OBJECTIVES TOWARD ACHIEVING A LONG-TERM GOAL

Long-Term Goal: Within 2 months, Matthew will improve sitting and standing balance so that he can dress himself independently.

Short-Term Behavioral Objectives:
1. Mathew will stand unassisted while conversing, for 1 min, 80% of the times requested.
2. During therapy, Matthew will maintain an upright sitting posture on the large therapy ball while being tilted side to side by the therapist for 20–30 sec.
3. In the morning, Matthew will get dressed while sitting on his bed, with minimal physical assistance for support in standing to pull up his pants and verbal cues, 80% of the time.

BOX 7-6	SAMPLE BEHAVIORAL OBJECTIVES TOWARD ACHIEVING A LONG-TERM GOAL

Long-Term Goal: By the end of the school year, Carol will improve her social skills so that she plays nicely with peers on the playground during recess.

Short-Term Objectives:

1. With verbal prompts, Carol initiates play with another classmate during free play time 50% of the time.

2. Carol will spontaneously initiate play with another classmate during free play time 80% of the time.

3. With assistance to follow the lead of others and take turns, Carol will participate in play successfully with peers during recess 50% of the time opportunities arise.

ences (parents, teachers, and physicians) can understand what you have written and your report is "professional." A professional report is clear, concise, and typewritten; contains no grammatical or spelling errors; is well organized; and contains accurate information. Standardized test scores should be reported and interpreted accurately, and your impressions, subjective interpretations, and recommendations should be clearly supported by the objective data that you include in your report (from results of standardized tests and from your observations). You should also take care to use politically correct language, such as person-first language (i.e., a child with autism instead of an autistic child), and to avoid negative language such as "inflicted with" or "suffers from." A standard length for writing evaluation reports has not been established, but most comprehensive reports can be completed in 3 to 6 typed pages.

Once your report has been written, it is important that you spend time with the child and family to go over the report and answer any questions that they may have. Typically, evaluation reports are sent to the referral source and to the family. They become part of the child's medical chart in a hospital setting and part of a child's official education record if the child was seen in an educational setting. Other team members or professionals working with the child outside of the setting you work in may also want a

(*Text continued on page 280*)

NORTHEAST PEDIATRIC THERAPY SERVICES
Occupational Therapy Initial Evaluation

Child's Name: *Pat B.*

DOB: *12/23/81*   **Age:** *15 years, 8 months*

Date of Evaluation: *September 17, 1997*

Parent Names, Address, Telephone: *Tony and Courtney B.*

Referral Source: *Pediatrician, Dr. A., mother initiated the referral*

Reason for Referral

Pat was referred for an occupational therapy evaluation to assist in determining whether sensory motor deficits were contributing to his behavioral concerns and academic difficulties at school. His mother was particularly interested in some assistance with identifying his educational needs and strategies for learning.

Methods of Evaluation

Pat was evaluated during a 11/2-hour session. He was brought to the clinic by his mother. Evaluation methods included:

- Parent and child interviews, which were conducted separately
- A nonstandardized sensorimotor history questionnaire completed by his mother
- Pat provided a handwriting sample
- Test of Visual-Motor Skills (Gardner), a design copy test was admininsterd
- Pat completed the Touch Inventory for Elementary School Children, a measure of tactile defensiveness
- Structured clinical observations of sensory processing, postural control, balance, coordination, gross motor skills, and computer play were conducted

Relevant Medical History and Occupational Profile

Pat was diagnosed with Attention-deficit hyperactivity disorder approximately 4 years ago and more recently with Asperger's syndrome and bipolar disorder. He is presently taking medication (Respiratol and Wellbutrin) for behavior management and is followed regularly by Dr. G., a child psychiatrist, for his mental health and medications. Pat's medical history is unremarkable for serious illness or hospitalizations. He is slightly taller and heavier than other 15-year-olds. Pat attends Rocky High School as a sophomore, where he receives educational programming from both general and special education. He has a full-time teacher's aide and two periods of study skills per day and weekly speech therapy. He reports that he likes school, and he is pleased about having the two extra periods of study skills because he can use this time to complete homework.

Pat is an only child and lives with his biological parents. They do not have extended family members in the immediate area, but his parents report that they have a close family and that Pat has good relationships with some of his cousins, aunts, uncles, and grandparents. The family lives in a rural area, in a neighborhood with many children. Pat was able to identify one friend that he sometimes hangs out

Figure 7–1. Sample initial evaluation report, clinic setting, adolescent.

Figure 7–1. (Continued)

with outside of school. As a family, they go on two or three short vacations a year, and they go to church on Sundays. Both mother and father work outside the home, and Pat can manage on his own after school. Currently, Pat does not participate in any organized groups, activities, or sports. He does do band at school, playing the trumpet, and enjoys watching TV, reading, and videogames. He also enjoys learning about cars and computers. He manages all of his basic self-care skills without difficulty and takes pride in his appearance. He does not have set chores around the house but likes to help his father with any mechanical-type home repairs.

Pat attended both physical and occupational therapy last year for a short time before relocating to this area. His previous occupational therapy evaluation, dated 12/30/1996, indicated sensory processing difficulties, including difficulties modulating sensory input (sometimes becoming easily overstimulated and other times being lethargic); poor postural control and poor physical endurance; and poor vestibular, tactile, and proprioceptive processing, which affected his performance in both the fine motor and gross motor areas. Physical therapy reports from the past year indicate decreased gross motor skills, hypotonia, decreased strength, and pronated feet.

Behavior During the Evaluation

Pat was pleasant and cooperative throughout the evaluation. He initiated little conversation; however, he answered all of my questions willingly and completely. He seemed somewhat anxious at times and frequently fidgeted with his hands. Eye contact was fleeting and overall affect was somewhat flat. He did smile and laugh appropriately. His activity level overall was on the low side. He tended to slump in his seat, and the quality of movements seemed slow and deliberate. His speech was also slow and deliberate, with an obvious lisp. He was slow to respond to questions, requiring an extra second or two during conversation to come up with a response. He also had on occasion what seemed to be word-finding difficulty. He was, however, able to stay on topic, and he displayed some sense of humor. He also concentrated well and seemed to put forth good effort on the standardized test that was given.

Child Interview and Results of the Touch Inventory

Pat reported that his main problem at school was his handwriting, which is a constant frustration for him. He also reported that his teacher's aide was with him all day for protection in case other kids beat him up. Apparently there had been previous incidents when he was threatened by other students. Pat also stated that his aide helps him be organized in his classes. Overall he stated that academics were going well and that school is a good way to pass the time. He reported that study skill periods helped him a great deal to get his homework done and that without them he probably would fall significantly behind in his schoolwork. He did not think that he would be disciplined enough to complete his homework at home. He described himself as a person with fluctuating moods, who tends to be more on the anxious side rather than the laid-back side, and somewhere in the middle of happy and sad. He said that the medication he is taking

Figure 7–1. *(Continued)*

helps him with self-control, levels his mood swings, reduces aggressive outbursts and impulsivity, and makes him overall more motivated and better able to concentrate.

Pat said that it is difficult for him to get along with others at times but that he has some friends and does not perceive social relationships as particularly troublesome. He reported that he knows his motor skills are poor but that he does OK and enjoys physical education at school and can manage everyday motor demands (getting to where he needs to go, getting dressed, etc.). He does not have any specific sport interests. He did report that he gets pain in both ankles, greater on the right side after walking for relatively short lengths of time (half hour). Results of the Touch Inventory indicated that Pat has no significant tactile hypersensitivities at this time. He did, however, report that some of the behaviors that indicate tactile hypersensitivity were behaviors that he exhibited in the past.

Parent Interview and Results of the Sensory History Questionnaire

His mom, Courtney, reported that her main concerns about Pat were related to the social and motor areas. In the social area, she has concerns about his ability to get along with others and develop friendships. In the motor area, she is most concerned about his handwriting, his motor clumsiness, and his lack of physical endurance. For example, she said "we go to the mall and we frequently have to stop and rest because Pat is too tired, and then he complains of pain in his ankles when he walks." She reported that the medication he is taking has been quite successful in managing his behavior. She is also concerned with respect to his emotional well-being and self-esteem. She feels that his educational programming has been effective, although she would like to see the amount of special education support he requires decrease.

The sensory history questionnaire completed by his mother is a series of questions asking the caregiver to rate the child's behavior on various items/behaviors that are believed to represent sensory processing abilities or problems. Her responses indicated that Pat does have some hypersensitivities to tactile (touch) input and that he is easily distracted by both auditory and visual sensory input. Problems were also evident in the vestibular/proprioceptive processing areas and affect the quality of his movements, balance and coordination, and physical endurance.

TVMS, Handwriting Sample, Computer Use

Normative data were not obtained for Pat on the TVMS, as children 12 years, 10 months is the highest group in which norms are available (approximately 2 years younger than his chronological age). He was, however, able to complete all designs accurately. He was notably shaky with the pencil, and he often drew his figures from left to right rather than right to left. His overall performance placed him somewhere above a motor age of 12 years, 10 months. Pat was asked to print a few sentences in response to four questions I posed. He did not complete the activity with complete sentences but responded with one- to three-word phrases. His printing was barely legible, with poor

Figure 7–1. *(Continued)*

spacing of letters and words. He made one letter reversal. Using the computer, he could type responses to the questions I posed much easier than writing them down. He did not use correct finger placement on the keyboard when typing, but he was very familiar with the location of the letters and demonstrated adequate dexterity to manage the mouse and keyboard. He could navigate the Internet and was proficient in managing the mouse and basic word-processing functions like using a spellcheck.

Clinical Observations

Pat was asked to perform a variety of motor activities, and his responses to a variety of sensory experiences were observed to evaluate sensory processing, basic postural and balance mechanisms, motor planning, strength, and coordination. Pat's muscle tone was globally minimally lowered, based on the lack of resistance felt on passive range of motion of the upper extremities and hyperextensibility of his joints. He experienced some difficulty with heel-to-toe walking, particularly with eyes closed. His balance reactions were present but slow to be elicited at times. Pat seemed to rely on visual cues rather than proprioceptive feedback to guide his balance. Pat could stand on one foot for greater than 10 sec, and he could hop on each foot about 10 times. He did these activities, however, with increased effort, and the quality of his movements again were compromised as they were slow and deliberate. Poor proprioceptive awareness was also evident during the finger-to-nose task where he was asked to touch his nose with his index fingers, with eyes closed. Movements were poorly graded and inaccurate. Pat could perform some jumping jacks. He could not skip, and attempts to teach him were unsuccessful. He also has flat feet, and, on weight bearing, his feet pronated bilaterally. He experienced difficulty coordinating both sides of his body together to perform smooth reciprocal movements. He reported that he never learned to ride a bike but that he never wanted to.

SUMMARY

The evaluation results indicate that Pat has some underlying sensory motor deficits that impact his daily life at home and school. More specifically, he demonstrates deficits with vestibular and proprioceptive processing, including low muscle tone, decreased balance, strength, and endurance; and incoordination. His problems are subtle, and he manages everyday motor tasks such as showering and mobility requirements at school. He reports that he manages alright in physical education at school. His leisure choices are, however, very sedentary, and endurance for walks (such as at the mall) is limiting. Of concern are reports of ankle pain after walking and significant pronation noted in both feet on weight bearing.

Fine motor performance is adequate for functional and leisure tasks such as computer play and dressing. However, he has difficulty with printing/handwriting, with his handwriting sample being more typical of a child in the second or third grade.

Some behavioral concerns were also evident and seem to be impacting his social relationships and feeling of self-worth and confidence. Interpretations based on my short time with him and his

Figure 7–1. *(Continued)*

mother, and from a review of relevant records, indicate that Pat has some difficulty maintaining and establishing peer relations and that his self-confidence and self-esteem are compromised. He seems to have few responsibilities and extracurricular activities in his life that allow him to gain self-confidence and a sense of achievement and that would provide opportunities to promote self-discipline, social skills, responsibility, and general independence. Based on parent and child reports, and my observations, his medication seems to be effective in managing his mood swings and aggression/self-control issues and in assisting with his ability to concentrate and organize his daily routine.

Pat was a pleasant young adolescent who displayed a good sense of humor when relaxed and given the opportunity to share stories of interest to him. With structure, encouragement, and some modifications, he has been successful in maintaining academic grades. Pat also has been able to identify some interests, including computers and cars. He seems to have a positive outlook despite the challenges that he faces every day in managing his behavior and compensating for his weaknesses with physical, motor coordination tasks.

Recommendations:

1. It seems that Pat has appropriate special education support and that his study skill periods are very helpful for him. His school special education and related service providers are best qualified to make specific recommendations regarding his education program. One suggestion to consider is to decrease the amount of time his aide is with him so that he be given more responsibility and is encouraged to attend some classes on his own. It is suspected that peer interactions may be limited simply because he has an adult with him a great deal of the time. Pat may also benefit from increased programming in the area of life skills such as money management, simple meal preparation, simple mechanics (as this is an area of interest for him), use of community resources, safety issues, etc.

2. It is recommended that Pat receive occupational therapy services at school to address his handwriting concerns and to explore alternative means for written communication, such as a laptop and perhaps voice recognition software. The school occupational therapist should also consult with the physical education teacher, to ensure that appropriate expectations are set for him in physical education. Finally, the occupational therapist may assist in addressing general environmental issues, including scheduling to maximize his ability to stay focused and organized and to reduce the risk of over-stimulation.

3. Short-term, clinic-based occupational therapy intervention is also recommended once per month for 4–5 months. Therapy goals would include exploring and trying out appropriate avenues to improve his motor coordination and physical endurance deficiencies and problem solving ways for Pat to compensate for his sensory motor challenges during functional activities. Pat, his mother, and I spoke about ways to promote his independence in the home

Figure 7–1. (Continued)

and the need to explore avenues to promote his leisure and social participation.

4. Orthopedic consult: Owing to reports of pain in his ankles, I feel it would be worthwhile for him to have an orthopedic consult to look more closely at a need for foot orthotics, including arch supports bilaterally.

It was a pleasure meeting Pat and his mother. If you have any questions or concerns regarding the information in this report, please feel free to contact me at 869-1122.

Sincerely,
Sue Martin, PhD, OTR/

Occupational Therapy Initial Evaluation

Name: Carly Z.

DOB: 2/5/92   **Age:** 8 years, 2 months

Test Dates: March 23, April 6, 2000

Grade: 2   **Teacher:** Mrs. Beatrice, 2/3 class

Reason for Referral

Carly was referred by her teacher for an occupational therapy evaluation and intervention because of reported fine and gross motor concerns. She is currently in a regular education, second-grade class and is being evaluated for the possible need for special education services.

Methods of Evaluation

Carly was evaluated during two 1-hour sessions. The Bruininks-Oseretsky Test of Motor Skills was administered to measure her fine and gross motor performance. Her parents completed the Sensory Profile (Dunn, 1999) to identify sensory processing concerns/abilities, and parent (both mother and father) and child informal interviews were conducted. Clinical observations of sensory processing, postural control, balance, coordination, and gross motor skills were also conducted as she played on the various pieces of therapy equipment. Classroom observations were also conducted during a small group, quiet work time, and her teacher was interviewed.

Relevant Medical History and Occupational Profile

Carly lives in a rural area, with her parents and twin sister, Cory, who has no reported developmental concerns. Carly was born 4 weeks early, at 5 lb, 10 oz, with no major complications. Her mother had uncomplicated gestational diabetes during pregnancy. Carly's medical history has been unremarkable, with no major illnesses or hospitalizations. She does, however, have a history of frequent ear infections. Her developmental milestones were reported to be achieved within the

Figure 7–2. Sample initial evaluation report, elementary school setting. (Continued)

Figure 7–2 (Continued)

age-appropriate ranges, and she was walking before 14 months of age. She was apparently a very fussy infant who was difficult to console.

Her mother reports that Carly was (and to some extent still is) a difficult child to raise. She states that Carly has difficulty following instructions, and it has been hard to know if it is because she is not listening, not processing the instructions, or noncompliant. She is easily distracted and often seems unaware of what is going on around her, although she seems to watch everything. For example, as a younger child, she needed to be watched very closely in parking lots because she sometimes would run out in front of a car. Her mother reports that she is a sensitive child who cries easily.

Carly had speech therapy when she was 4–5 years of age and has had some counseling services. She currently takes swimming lessons and she has taken ballet classes in the past. Her mother reported that as a young child, Carly preferred sedentary activities and avoided play on playground equipment. However, currently, despite a reported weakness with gross skills, she enjoys gross motor activity and seems fearless and sometimes unsafe as she plays. She gets along well with her sister. Carly enjoys school, especially art, and science.

Behavior During My Interview, Administration of the Bruininks-Oseretsky, and Clinical Observations

Carly was pleasant and cooperative throughout the evaluation. She was very friendly and talkative...almost excessively considering I was an unfamiliar adult. She seemed very comfortable with an unfamiliar person. She required encouragement at times to persist when challenged, and she was somewhat distracted by the abundance of visual stimuli in the therapy room. Her activity level overall was slightly higher than one would expect, although she could settle nicely at the table to perform fine motor, and pencil activities. She rarely stayed with the same activity more than 2–3 min unless coaxed to do so. She could carry on a conversation, although she tended to ramble on at times. She was overly affectionate at times, and liked to give hugs. She seemed to be a happy child who was eager to please and who often wanted feedback about how she was doing. She could follow directions well, and the test results are believed to reflect her true abilities.

Assessment Results:

The Sensory Profile, a parent questionnaire, was completed by her mother. The results revealed that Carly processes and modulates sensory information from the visual, auditory, vestibular, and tactile (touch) systems in many atypical ways. Specific scores are presented below. "Typical" scores are those that fall within 1 SD of the mean; scores interpreted as being in the "Probable Difference" range are scores between 1 and 2 SD below the mean; scores in the "Definite Difference" range are scores more than 2 SD below the mean.

Section	Raw Score	Interpretation
Auditory processing	25/40	Definite difference; easily distracted by auditory stimulation
Visual processing	31/45	Probable difference; poor figure-ground discrimination; puzzles are hard for her

Figure 7–2 (Continued)

Section	Raw Score	Interpretation
Vestibular processing	39/55	Definite difference; fear of heights; seeks movement like fidgeting; tends to be "on the go"
Touch processing	62/90	Definite difference; subtle hyper-sensitivity; dislikes grooming activities; touches others/objects excessively
Multisensory processing	20/35	Definite difference; decreased attention
Oral Sensory processing	46/60	Typical performance
Modulation endurance/tone	29/25	Definite difference; weak mus-cles; poor endurance
Modulation related to body position and movement	31/50	Definite difference; seems acci-dent prone

Section	Raw Score	Interpretation
Movement affecting activity	26/35	Typical; may become overly excitable during movement activity
Modulation of sensory input affecting emotional response	20-Nov	Definite difference; needs more protection than other children; can be overly affectionate
Modulation of visual input affecting emo-tional response/activity level	20-Dec	Probable difference (1–2 SD below the norm)
Emotional/social response	58/85	Probable difference; is sensitive to criticism and often expresses feelings of failure
Behavioral outcomes	18/30	Definite difference; poor fine motor skill
Thresholds for response	15-Oct	Probable difference; tends to jump frequently from activity to activity

In summary, Carly performed in the definite difference range in 8 of 14 areas, indicating that she processes and modulates sensory infor-mation in ways that are atypical compared with other children. Carly has some subtle hypersensitivities to auditory and tactile sensory information. Despite this hypersensitivity, she does seek sensory information (particularly from touch and movement) to help her explore and learn and perhaps as a means to calm herself. Carly touches others excessively at times, can be easily overexcited, and seeks movement experiences. When she is in control of the situation, she easily tolerates the sensory stimulation and tends to seek it out.

Figure 7–2 *(Continued)*

Behaviors reflective of low muscle tone and decreased physical endurance were identified. In the visual area, she experiences difficulty with figure-ground discrimination, and visual perceptual tasks such as putting puzzles together are difficult for her. Carly was described as a child whose self-esteem is fragile and who experiences difficulty relating to her peers and adapting to changes in routine. Factor scores consistent with this profile indicated that she has low endurance/tone and that she tends to be sensory seeking, and emotionally reactive, with decreased attention and distractibility.

Results of the Bruininks-Oseretsky Test of Motor Proficiency were as follows:

Gross Motor Subtests	Standard Score (Mean=15, SD=5)	Age Equiv. Sc
Running speed	6, below average	5 years, 11 months
Balance	6, below average	5 years, 5 months
Bilateral coordination	8, below average	5 years, 11 months
Strength	12, low average	6 years, 11 months
Gross Motor Composite Standard Score: 30, 2nd percentile		

Gross Motor Subtests	Standard Score (Mean=15, SD=5)	Age Equiv. Sc
Upper-limb coordination	8, below average	6 years, 2 months
Fine Motor Subtests		
Response speed	10, below average	6 years, 2 months
Visual-motor control	18, high average	9 years, 2 months
Upper-limb speed/dexterity	17, average	8 years, 2 months
Fine Motor Composite Standard Score: 51, 54th percentile		

Therefore, Carly demonstrated weaknesses in all areas of gross motor function. In the strength area, she experienced difficulty performing sit-ups (did 10 in 20 sec) and knee push-ups (she did 4). Her running gait was somewhat awkward, without smooth reciprocal arm and leg movements. She experienced difficulty walking on the balance beam and maintaining her balance with vision occluded. It was also noted that she watches her body carefully when she is moving. This indicates that Carly relies more on her visual skills to help orient her rather than her sense of proprioception and to produce coordinated motor movements. She also demonstrated difficulties coordinating both sides of her body together to catch a tennis ball, to perform various jumping sequences, and to complete foot and finger tapping patterns.

Carly performed well on the 2/3 fine motor tests, including items such as a tracing-type activity, design copy, cutting with scissors, and manipulating small objects such as pennies and pegs quickly. Carly was very motivated during these activities, and despite her good performance, she seemed to expend a great deal of energy doing so.

Figure 7–2 (Continued)

Clinical Observations:

I observed Carly perform a variety of motor activities and her responses to different forms of sensory input to evaluate sensory processing, basic postural and balance mechanisms, motor planning, strength, and coordination. Carly's muscle tone was globally minimally lowered, based on palpation of the muscle bellies and lack of resistance during passive range of movement of the upper extremities. Her movements at times were poorly graded and inaccurate. Carly could stand on one foot for greater than 10 sec, and could hop on each foot about 10 times. However, she did these activities with increased effort, and the quality of her movements again were compromised, as they were very deliberate. She experienced some difficulty coordinating both sides of her body together to perform smooth reciprocal movements. These difficulties collectively indicate a weakness with vestibular processing. It was also noted that Carly was somewhat impulsive on the equipment, with little appreciation for safety at times. She was, however, able to respond consistently to verbal cues to slow down and "think before doing."

Carly could motor plan adequately, as she could imitate simple and complex postures and motor sequences. However, when the motor sequences required a great deal of bilateral integration and were greater than five steps, she experienced much more difficulty. Carly could figure out how to play on various pieces of novel therapy equipment. Carly engaged in a great deal of sensory-seeking behavior. She explored the therapy room and had a hard time settling in to select a particular activity and then stick with it. She did not demonstrate any tactile hypersensitivities (played in the ball tunnel; played in the bucket of beans, Playdough, etc.), and she tolerated my physical handling well. Socially, she was a bit invasive at times, without appreciation for my personal space. Her energy level was slightly higher than one would expect despite clear fatigue/endurance limitations when physically challenged.

Classroom Observations:

Carly was observed in her classroom. Her classroom is a busy environment with a lot of artwork on the walls and hanging from the ceiling and a wall of windows facing the playground. Desks were arranged in groups of four, and there were two desks in one corner at the back of the room and a small couch. Carly was sitting with three classmates and they were working on completing two math sheets consisting of money problems. There were coins for each cluster of tables to assist them. Carly was working well, occasionally talking with her peers, and working toward completing her sheet. She rarely sat down, choosing to stand rather than sit. A few other children were also doing this. When seated, Carly moved frequently in her seat and seemed uncomfortable. Her sitting posture was poor. She rarely sat up straight, and she tended to keep her head lying on the table or very close to the page. The teacher and one other adult, a volunteer, were in the room. The volunteer was moving around and helping the children while the teacher stayed at her desk. On one occasion, Carly got up to tell the teacher something, and the teacher listened briefly and then asked her to go back and sit down. On two occasions, the teacher asked the children to quiet down and reduce the noise level in the room. Carly seemed to enjoy handling the money. She was actively involved in figuring out the problems, although she did not always print the written answers on her work sheet. The written work she did produce was com-

Figure 7–2 *(Continued)*

parable to that of the other children, and she used a mature tripod pencil grasp on her pencil. When the 15 min was up, Carly had completed one of the sheets but not the second. Most of the other children had completed or nearly completed the second sheet. The children were then asked to put their work away, get ready for recess, and line up. Carly was ordering the other children in her group to help and seemed to take charge of the cleanup effort. The other children seemed a little annoyed at this. She was one of the last children to get into line to go out for recess.

Her teacher reported that Carly is keeping up with the academic demands of second grade so far but that she needs more cues to keep focused and more encouragement than the other children. She tends to work slowly and needs to move around during the school day more than the other children. Socially, she has a few friends in the class but often is loud and bossy. On the other hand, she relates to teachers well and is very clingy at times. She experiences some difficulty keeping up with the others in physical education and does not like it.

SUMMARY

Evaluation data from standardized testing, clinical and classroom observations, and informal interviews indicate that Carly has some sensory and motor deficits that impact her daily life and school performance in some areas. She is compromised in areas of vestibular and proprioceptive processing, which impact her balance, coordination, and overall gross motor skills. She is also easily distracted by both visual and auditory sensory stimuli, and overall she tends to engage in sensory-seeking behavior. Her gross motor skills are approximately 1 year delayed, and her fine motor skills were assessed to within normal limits. Her gross motor limitations impacted her performance in physical education at school.

Some behavioral concerns (although mild) were also evident and impact her functioning. Carly is somewhat impulsive and easily distracted. She experiences difficulty following directions at times and organizing herself to complete tasks. She also can be somewhat invasive socially (little regard for personal space). However, Carly is a fun, friendly, and compassionate individual who works hard to please others. With frequent teacher contact and encouragement she has been successful in school-related activities.

Recommendations:

1. Based on her gross motor test scores, Carly is eligible for occupational therapy services provided she qualifies for a special education coding. It is recommended that Carly receive occupational therapy services at school to address her sensory and motor challenges, as they are impacting her performance in physical education, her ability to organize and complete school assignments, and her ability to develop satisfying peer relationships. For example, strategies can be developed to help her compensate for her tactile and auditory hypersensitivities and sensory-seeking behavior and to reduce the negative impact they have on her performance in the classroom. Opportunities for her to develop gross motor skills, including improving her balance and increasing her muscle strength, postural control, and bilateral coordination, should also be part of her educational program as well as consulting with physical education teachers to ensure that she has a more positive experience. A specific plan, including scheduling and writing goals and objectives, will be developed at an upcoming meeting.

Figure 7–2 (Continued)

2. Some suggestions for the home include the following: Carly is currently taking swimming lessons, and this is believed to be a good activity for her if she enjoys it. All physical activity to improve general strength and endurance, balance, and coordination would be good for her. Individual sports are suggested rather than competitive team sports, which may result in frustration. For example, bike riding, tennis, roller blading, jumping on a trampoline, dance, and hiking are a few suggestions.

3. Carly is a child who seeks sensory input; therefore, she should be provided with a lot of opportunities to engage in activities rich in multisensory input. Hands-on learning opportunities, craft projects, time to run around, etc., would be good for her. Also, during times when she must be more focused, give her a little time to prepare so she knows that she needs to slow down, think, and attend. Having her repeat directions is a good habit to get into to ensure that she has processed what has been asked of her.

I can be reached at 899-1122 if you have any questions about the information in this report.

Sue Kelly, MS, OTR/L

Occupational Therapy Initial Evaluation Report

Child's Name: *Hannah N.*

Date of Birth: *May 5, 1999*   **Age:** *3 years, 6 months*

Parent/Legal Guardian Names: *Jan N.*

Date(s) of Evaluation: *November 5, 2002*

Referring Information: (See the chart for medical history and details of injuries sustained in the motor vehicle accident). Hannah was involved in a motor vehicle accident on October 8 of this year in which she was a pedestrian. The accident resulted in a severe traumatic brain injury, and she was transferred from intensive care to acute care this week. She currently is medically stable, although she is on constant respiratory and cardiac monitoring as a precaution and is tube fed. Diagnostic testing revealed diffuse encephalopathy with enlarged ventricles, with more disturbance in the right frontal and occipital areas and postparietal regions. Reports indicate that, to date, she has not regained consciousness, although she has opened her eyes and exhibits some spontaneous movement.

Evaluation Methods: Functional bedside evaluation with physical therapist, Comprehensive Level of Consciousness Scale (CLOCS), interviews with nursing and mother

Child's Occupational Profile: Hannah lives with her mother, who is a single parent, and her 6-year-old brother. Her biological father is not involved in her care. Before the accident, Hannah attended a full-time center-based day care program while her mother worked as a

Figure 7–3. Sample initial evaluation report, hospital, acute care, toddler. (*Continued*)

Figure 7–3 *(Continued)*

store manager. Her medical history before the accident was unremarkable, and she was developing normally. She enjoys playing with the children at the day care and with her brother, and she is particularly interested in music and dancing. Her mother is coping as well as can be expected. She reports feeling helpless and would like to be able to do more for her daughter. She has been given a leave of absence from work, and spends most of her days at the hospital with her daughter.

Evaluation Results: Hannah did not respond to verbal requests or to her name, and she kept her eyes closed for the 30 min we evaluated her. Her score on the CLOCS was very low, at 13. She did not make any vocalizations; there was no spontaneous eye opening or pupillary light reflexes, and her response to noxious stimuli was a weak disorganized withdrawal (see form in chart for details). She is fully dependent with all self-care needs and is tube fed. She exhibits full upper-extremity and lower-extremity range of motion. Muscle tone was assessed to be moderately increased in the lower extremities and right extremity, and she is at risk for losing range of motion. Some weak, spontaneous movement of all four limbs was noted, although not purposeful. Nursing reports that she is able to tolerate a supported, semireclined sitting position for up to about 30 min.

Evaluation Summary and Impressions: Hannah's recovery to date has been slow, and she has not regained consciousness. Although she exhibits little spontaneous movement and increased muscle tone, she has maintained full range of motion of her limbs. Her response to stimuli is limited to a gross, disorganized withdrawal. Her mother has been extremely supportive and is motivated to do all that she can for her daughter.

Recommendations: Hannah is not yet ready for active rehabilitation. She will, however be seen 5 times per week for cognitive stimulation and to monitor her level of consciousness, passive and active range of motion as she is able, and positioning concerns and for parent support as needed. Activities of daily living training, including functional mobility and feeding, will begin once her level of consciousness improves.

Molly F. OTR/L

copy of your evaluation report. With the parents' written consent, you can send a copy to them as well.

Often you may be asked to report your evaluation findings in the context of a team meeting in early-intervention, educational, or hospital settings. It is important to be able to summarize your major findings and recommendations in about 3 to 5 minutes. When **reporting your findings**, it is important

Child's Name:

Date of Birth: Age:

Parent/Legal Guardian Names:

Address and Telephone Number:

Date(s) of Evaluation:

Educational Program: (name of school, grade, type of school program, teacher's name

Referring Information: (referral source, reasons for referral, child's primary physician)

Evaluation Methods: (provide a brief description of the assessment methods and any standardized tests used)

Child's Occupational Profile: (relevant background information, including medical history, presenting problems, valued activities, and relationships)

Behavior During the Evaluation: (summarize the child's behavior during the assessment and include a statement of how the child's behavior may have influenced any test results)

Evaluation Results: (include test scores and clinical observations)

Evaluation Summary and Impressions: (synthesis and summary of all the evaluation information, including the child's strengths and challenges)

Recommendations:

Your name, signature, and qualifications and contact telephone number

Figure 7–4. Occupational therapy initial evaluation report.

to summarize what you did during your evaluation. Highlight the major findings, including summarizing test scores; the child strengths, challenges, and needs; and how the child's difficulties impact his or her ability to participate in valued occupations (roles and activities). Finally, briefly describe what your intentions are for further involvement, including any recommendations for occupational therapy intervention.

SUMMARY

This chapter expanded on information on the final three steps of the evaluation process presented in Chapter 2 and emphasized methods of synthesizing evaluation data for intervention planning, writing goals, and communicating evaluation results through report writing. Synthesizing and summarizing evaluation data and the intervention planning that follows are probably the most challenging clinical activities that you will engage in as an occupational therapist. Your proficiency in completing these steps for individual clients will continue to evolve throughout your years as a practitioner. The content of this book does not include information regarding the intervention process or specific intervention techniques. It is, however, important to point out that your knowledge and skills related to intervention play an important role in determining what your intervention programs will ultimately look like. Collaborating with others, especially the child and parents, the importance of making discharge projections or identifying long-term functional goals, and of applying the best available research were highlighted as essential considerations throughout the intervention planning process, regardless of practice setting. Guidelines for writing intervention goals and behavioral objectives and for creating evaluation reports were also included, with examples.

References

American Occupational Therapy Association (2002). The Occupational Therapy Practice Framework: Author.

Individuals with Disabilities Education Act (IDEA) Amendments of 1997 (PL.105-17). U.S.C. 1400.

Sackett, D.L., Rosenberg, W.M., Gray, J., Haynes, R., & Richardson, W.S. (1996). Evidence-based medicine: What it is and what it isn't. *British Medical Journal, 312,* 71–72.

Zimmerman, J. (1988). *Goals and objectives for developing normal movement patterns.* Rockville, MD: Aspen Publishing.

A

Excerpts From the American Occupational Therapy Association's *Occupational Therapy Practice Framework* Related to Evaluation

The text in this appendix has been reprinted with permission from the Commission on Practice, American Occupational Therapy Association. *Occupational Therapy Practice Framework*. Available at: http://www.aota.org. 2002.

EVALUATION PROCESS

The evaluation process sets the stage for all that follows. Because occupational therapy is concerned with performance in daily life and how performance affects engagement in occupations to support participation, the evaluation process is focused on finding out what the client wants and needs to do and on identifying those factors that act as supports or barriers to performance. During the evaluation process, this information is paired with the occupational therapist's knowledge about human performance and the effect that illness, disability, and engagement in occupation have on performance. The occupational therapist considers performance skills, performance patterns, context, activity demands, and client factors and determines how each influences performance. The occupational therapist's skilled observation, use of specific assessments, and interpretation of results leads to a clear delineation of the problems and probable causes. The occupational therapy assistant may contribute to the evaluation process based on established competencies and under the supervision of an occupational therapist.

During the evaluation, a collaborative relationship with the client is established that continues throughout the entire occupational therapy process. The evaluation process is divided into two substeps: the occupational profile and analysis of occupational performance. The occupational profile is the initial step during which the client's needs, problems, and concerns about occupations and daily life activity performance are identified and priorities and values are ascertained. The client's background and history in reference to engagement in occupations and in activities are also explored. The second substep of the evaluation process, analysis of occupational performance, focuses on more specifically identifying occupational performance issues and evaluating selected factors that support and hinder performance. Although each substep is described separately and sequentially, in actuality, information pertinent to both substeps may be gathered during either one. The client's input is central in this process, and the client's priorities guide choices and decisions made during the process of evaluation.

Occupational Profile

An occupational profile is defined as information that describes the client's occupational history and experiences, patterns of daily living, interests, values, and needs. The profile is designed to gain an understanding of the client's perspective and background. Using a client-centered approach, information is gathered to understand what is currently important and meaningful to the client (what he or she wants and needs to do) and to identify past experiences and interests that may assist in the understanding of current issues and problems. During the process of collecting this information, the client's priorities and desired targeted outcomes that will lead to engagement in occupation to support participation in life are also identified. Only clients can identify the occupations that give meaning to their lives and select the goals and priorities that are important to them. Valuing and respecting the client's input helps to foster client involvement and can more efficiently guide interventions. Information about the occupational profile is collected at the beginning of contact with the client. However, additional information is collected over time throughout the process, refined, and reflected in changes subsequently made to targeted outcomes.

Process (Related to Developing the Occupational Profile)

The theories and frames of reference that the occupational therapist selects to guide his or her reasoning will influence the information that is collected during the occupational profile. Scientific knowledge and evidence about diagnostic conditions and occupational performance problems is used to guide information gathering.

The process of completing the occupational profile will vary depending on the setting and the client. The information gathered in the profile may be obtained both formally and informally and may be completed in one session or over a much longer period while working with the client. Obtaining information through both formal interview and casual conversation is a way of beginning to establish a therapeutic relationship with the client. Ideally, the information obtained through the occupational profile will lead to a more individualized approach in the evaluation, intervention planning, and intervention implementation stages. Specifically, the following information is collected:

- Who is the client (individual, caregiver, group, population)?
- Why is the client seeking service, and what are the client's current concerns relative to engaging in occupations and in daily life activities?
- What areas of occupation are successful, and what areas are causing problems or risks?
- What contexts support engagement in desired occupations, and what contexts are inhibiting engagement?
- What is the client's occupational history (i.e., life experiences, values, interests, previous patterns of

engagement in occupations and in daily life activities, the meanings associated with them)?
- What are the client's priorities and desired targeted outcomes (see AOTA Practice Framework Appendix, Table 9)? –Occupational performance –Client satisfaction–Role competence–Adaptation –Health and wellness –Prevention –Quality of life

After profile data are collected, the therapist reviews the information and develops a working hypothesis regarding possible reasons for identified problems and concerns and identifies the client's strengths and weaknesses. Outcome measures are preliminarily selected.

Analysis of Occupational Performance

Occupational performance is defined as the ability to carry out activities of daily life, including activities in the areas of occupation: activities of daily living (ADLs) (also called basic ADLs and personal ADLs), instrumental ADLs, education, work, play, leisure, and social participation. Occupational performance results in accomplishment of the selected occupation or activity and occurs through a dynamic transaction among the client, the context, and the activity. Improving or developing skills and patterns in occupational performance leads to engagement in one or more occupations (adapted in part from Law et al., 1996, p. 16). When occupational performance is analyzed, the performance skills and patterns used in performance are identified, and other aspects of engaging in occupation that affect skills and patterns (e.g., client factors, activity demands, and context or contexts) are evaluated. The analysis process identifies facilitators as well as barriers in various aspects of engagement in occupations and in ADLs. Analyzing occupational performance requires an understanding of the complex and dynamic interaction among performance skills, performance patterns, context or contexts, activity demands, and client factors rather than of any one factor alone. The information gathered during the occupational profile about the client's needs, problems, and priorities guides decisions during the analysis of occupational performance. The profile information directs the therapist's selection of the specific occupations or activities that need to be further analyzed and influences the selection of specific assessments that are used during the analysis process.

Process (Related to the Analysis of Occupational Performance)

Using available evidence and all aspects of clinical reasoning (scientific, narrative, pragmatic, and ethical), the therapist selects one or more frames of reference to guide further collection of evaluation information. The following actions are taken:

- Synthesize information from the occupational profile to focus on specific areas of occupation and their contexts that need to be addressed.
- Observe the client's performance in desired occupations and activities, noting effectiveness of the performance skills and performance patterns. May select and use specific assessments to measure performance skills and patterns as appropriate.
- Select assessments, as needed, to identify and measure more specifically context or contexts, activity demands, and client factors that may be influencing performance skills and performance patterns.
- Interpret the assessment data to identify what supports performance and what hinders performance.
- Develop and refine hypotheses about the client's occupational performance strengths and weaknesses.
- Create goals in collaboration with the client that address the desired targeted outcomes. Confirm outcome measure to be used.
- Delineate a potential intervention approach or approaches based on best practice and evidence.

INTERVENTION PROCESS

The intervention process is divided into three substeps: intervention plan, intervention implementation, and intervention review. During the intervention process, information from the evaluation step is integrated with theory, frames of reference, and evidence and is coupled with clinical reasoning to develop a plan and carry it out. The plan guides the actions of the occupational therapist and occupational therapy assistant and is based on the client's priorities.

BOX A-1	AREAS OF OCCUPATION

(Various kinds of life activities in which people engage, including ADLs, IADLs, education, work, play, leisure, and social participation.)

Activities of daily living (ADLs)—Activities that are oriented toward taking care of one's own body (adapted from Rogers and Holm, 1994, pp. 181–202)—also called basic ADLs or personal ADLs.

- *Bathing, showering*—Obtaining and using supplies; soaping, rinsing, and drying body parts; maintaining bathing position; and transferring to and from bathing positions.

- *Bowel and bladder management*—Includes complete intentional control of bowel movements and urinary bladder and, if necessary, use of equipment or agents for bladder control (Uniform Data System for Medical Rehabilitation [UDSMR], 1996, pp. III-20, III-24).

- *Dressing*—Selecting clothing and accessories appropriate to time of day, weather, and occasion; obtaining clothing from storage area; dressing and undressing in a sequential fashion; fastening and adjusting clothing and shoes; prostheses, or orthoses.

- *Eating*—"The ability to keep and manipulate food/fluid in the mouth and swallow it (O'Sullivan, 1995, p. 191)" (AOTA, 2000, p. 629).

- *Feeding*—"The process of setting up, arranging, and bringing food [fluids] from the plate or cup to the mouth (O'Sullivan, 1995, p. 191)" (AOTA, 2000, p. 629).

- *Functional mobility*—Moving from one position or place to another (during performance of everyday activities), such as in-bed mobility, wheelchair mobility, and transfers (wheelchair, bed, car, tub, toilet, shower, chair, floor). Performing functional ambulation and transporting objects.

- *Personal device care*—Using, cleaning, and maintaining personal care items, such as hearing aids, contact lenses, glasses, orthoses, prostheses, adaptive equipment, and contraceptive and sexual devices.

- *Personal hygiene and grooming*—Obtaining and using supplies; removing body hair (use of razors, tweezers, lotions, etc.); applying and removing cosmetics; washing, drying, combing, styling,

BOX A-1	AREAS OF OCCUPATION

caring for skin, ears, eyes, and nose; applying deodorant; cleaning mouth; and brushing and flossing teeth or removing, cleaning, and reinserting dental orthoses and prostheses.

- *Sexual activity*—Engagement in activities that result in sexual satisfaction.

- *Sleep/rest*—A period of inactivity in which one may or may not suspend consciousness.

- *Toilet hygiene*—Obtaining and using supplies; clothing management; maintaining toileting position; transferring to and from toileting position; cleaning body; and caring for menstrual and continence needs (including catheters, colostomies, and suppository management).

Instrumental activities of daily living (IADLs)—Activities that are oriented toward interacting with the environment and that are often complex and generally optional in nature (i.e., may be delegated to another) (adapted from Rogers and Holm, 1994, pp. 181–202).

- *Care of others* (including selecting and supervising caregivers)—Arranging, supervising, or providing the care for others.

- *Care of pets*—Arranging, supervising, or providing the care for pets and service animals.

- *Child rearing*—Providing the care and supervision to support the developmental needs of a child.

- *Communication device use*—Using equipment or systems such as writing equipment, telephones, typewriters, computers, communication boards, call lights, emergency systems, braille writers, telecommunication devices for the deaf, and augmentative communication systems to send and receive information.

- *Community mobility*—Moving self in the community and using public or private transportation, such as driving, or accessing buses, taxicabs, or other public transportation systems.

- *Financial management*—Using fiscal resources, including alternate methods of financial transaction and planning and using finances with long-term and short-term goals.

- *Health management and maintenance*—Developing, managing, and maintaining routines for health and wellness promotion, such as physical fitness, nutrition, decreasing health risk behaviors, and medication routines.

- *Home establishment and management*—Obtaining and maintaining personal and household possessions and environment (e.g., home, yard, garden, appliances, and vehicles), including maintaining and repairing personal possessions

(continued)

BOX A-1	AREAS OF OCCUPATION *(Continued)*

(clothing and household items) and knowing how to seek help or whom to contact.

- *Meal preparation and cleanup*—Planning, preparing, and serving well-balanced, nutritional meals and cleaning up food and utensils after meals.

- *Safety procedures and emergency responses*—Knowing and performing preventive procedures to maintain a safe environment as well as recognizing sudden, unexpected hazardous situations and initiating emergency action to reduce the threat to health and safety.

- *Shopping*—Preparing shopping lists (grocery and other), selecting and purchasing items, selecting method of payment, and completing money transactions.

Education—Includes activities needed for being a student and participating in a learning environment.

- *Formal educational participation*—Including the categories of academic (e.g., math, reading, working on a degree), nonacademic (e.g., recess, lunchroom, hallway), extracurricular (e.g., sports, band, cheerleading, dances), and vocational (prevocational and vocational) participation.

- *Exploration of informal personal educational needs or interests* (beyond formal education)—Identifying topics and methods for obtaining topic-related information or skills.

- *Informal personal education participation*—Participating in classes, programs, and activities that provide instruction/training in identified areas of interest.

Work—Includes activities needed for engaging in remunerative employment or volunteer activities (Mosey, 1996, pp. 341).

- *Employment interests and pursuits*—Identifying and selecting work opportunities based on personal assets, limitations, likes, and dislikes relative to work (adapted from Mosey, 1996, p. 342).

- *Employment seeking and acquisition*—Identifying job opportunities, completing and submitting appropriate application materials, preparing for interviews, participating in interviews and following up afterward, discussing job benefits, and finalizing negotiations.

- *Job performance*—Including work habits, e.g., attendance, punctuality, appropriate relationships with coworkers and supervisors, completion of assigned work, and compliance with the norms of the work setting (adapted from Mosey, 1996, p. 342).

- *Retirement preparation and adjustment*—Determining aptitudes, developing interests and skills, and selecting appropriate avocational pursuits.

BOX A-1	AREAS OF OCCUPATION *(Continued)*

- *Volunteer exploration*—Determining community causes, organizations, or opportunities for unpaid "work" in relationship to personal skills, interests, location, and time available.

- *Volunteer participation*—Performing unpaid "work" activities for the benefit of identified selected causes, organizations, or facilities.

Play—"Any spontaneous or organized activity that provides enjoyment, entertainment, amusement, or diversion" (Parham and Fazio, 1997, p. 252).

- *Play exploration*—Identifying appropriate play activities, which can include exploration play, practice play, pretend play, games with rules, constructive play, and symbolic play (adapted from Bergen, 1988, pp. 64-65).

- *Play participation*—Participating in play; maintaining a balance of play with other areas of occupation; and obtaining, using, and maintaining, toys, equipment, and supplies appropriately.

Leisure—"A nonobligatory activity that is intrinsically motivated and engaged in during discretionary time, that is time not committed to obligatory occupations such as work, self-care or sleep"(Parham and Fazio, p. 250).

- *Leisure exploration*—Identifying interests, skills, opportunities, and appropriate leisure activities.

- *Leisure participation*—Planning and participating in appropriate leisure activities; maintaining a balance of leisure activities with other areas of occupation; and obtaining, using, and maintaining equipment and supplies as appropriate.

Social participation—Activities associated with organized patterns of behavior that are characteristic and expected of an individual or an individual interacting with others within a given social system (adapted from Mosey, 1996, p. 340).

- *Community*—Activities that result in successful interaction at the community level (i.e., neighborhood, organizations, work, school).

- *Family*—"[Activities that result in] successful interaction in specific required and/or desired familial roles" (Mosey, 1996, p. 340).

- *Peer, friend*—Activities at different levels of intimacy, including engaging in desired sexual activity.

Some of the terms used in this table are from, or are adapted from, the rescinded *Uniform Terminology for Occupational Therapy*—Third Edition (AOTA, 1994, pp. 1047–1054).

BOX A-2	PERFORMANCE SKILLS

Features of what one does, not what one has, related to observable elements of action that have implicit functional purposes (adapted from Fisher and Kielhofner, 1995, p.113).

Motor skills—Skills in moving and interacting with tasks, objects, and environment (A. Fisher, personal communication, July 9, 2001).

- *Posture*—Relates to the stabilizing and aligning of one's body while moving in relation to task objects with which one must deal.

    Stabilizes—Maintains trunk control and balance while interacting with task objects such that there is no evidence of transient (i.e., quickly passing) propping or loss of balance that affects task performance.

    Aligns—Maintains an upright sitting or standing position without evidence of a need to persistently prop during the task performance.

    Positions—Positions body, arms, or wheelchair in relation to task objects and in a manner that promotes the use of efficient arm movement performance.

- *Mobility*—Relates to moving the entire body or a body part in space as necessary when interacting with task objects.

    Walks—Ambulates on level surfaces and changes direction while walking without shuffling the feet, lurching, instability, or using external supports or assistive devices (e.g., cane, walker).

    Reaches—Extends, moves the arm (and when appropriate, the trunk) to effectively grasp or place task objects that are out of reach, including skillfully using a reacher to obtain task objects.

    Bends—Actively flexes, rotates, or twists the trunk in a manner and direction appropriate to the task.

- *Coordination*—Relates to using more than one body part to interact with task objects in a manner that supports task performance.

    Coordinates—Uses two or more body parts together to stabilize and manipulate task objects during bilateral motor tasks.

    Manipulates—Uses dexterous grasp-and-release patterns, isolated finger movements, and coordinated in-hand manipulation patterns when interacting with task objects.

    Flows—Uses smooth and fluid arm and hand movements when interacting with task objects.

- *Strength and effort*—Pertains to skills that require generation of muscle force appropriate for effective interaction with task objects.

    Moves—Pushes, pulls, or drags task objects along a supporting surface.

BOX A-2	PERFORMANCE SKILLS

Transports—Carries task objects from one place to another while walking, seated in a wheelchair, or using a walker.

Lifts—Raises or hoists task objects, including lifting an object from one place to another, but without ambulating or moving from one place to another.

Calibrates—Regulates or grades the force speed and extent of movement when interacting with task objects (e.g., not too much or too little).

Grips—Pinches or grasps task objects with no "grip slips."

- *Energy*—Refers to sustained effort over the course of task performance.

  Endures—Persists and completes the task without obvious evidence of physical fatigue, pausing to rest, or stopping to "catch one's breath."

  Paces—Maintains a consistent and effective rate or tempo of performance throughout the steps of the entire task.

Process skills—"Skills...used in managing and modifying actions en route to the completion of daily life tasks" (Fisher and Kielhofner, p. 120).

- *Energy*—Refers to sustained effort over the course of task performance.

  Paces—Maintains a consistent and effective rate or tempo of performance throughout the steps of the entire task.

  Attends—Maintains focused attention throughout the task such that the client is not distracted away from the task by extraneous auditory or visual stimuli.

- *Knowledge*—Refers to the ability to seek and use task-related knowledge.

  Chooses—Selects appropriate and necessary tools and materials for the task, including choosing the tools and materials that were specified for use before initiation of the task.

  Uses—Uses tools and materials according to their intended purposes and in a reasonable or hygienic fashion given their intrinsic properties and the availability (or lack of availability) of other objects.

  Handles—Supports, stabilizes, and holds tools and materials in an appropriate manner that protects them from damage, falling, or dropping.

(continued)

| BOX A-2 | PERFORMANCE SKILLS *(Continued)* |

Heeds—Uses goal-directed task actions that are focused toward the completion of the specified task (i.e., the outcome originally agreed on or specified by another) without behavior that is driven or guided by environmental cues (i.e., "environmentally cued behavior").

Inquires—Seeks needed verbal or written information by asking questions or reading directions or labels or asks no unnecessary information questions (e.g., questions related to where materials are located or how a familiar task is performed).

- *Temporal organization*—Pertains to the beginning, logical ordering, continuation, and completion of the steps and action sequences of a task.

  Initiates—Starts or begins the next action or step without hesitation.

  Continues—Performs actions or action sequences of steps without unnecessary interruption such that once an action sequence is initiated, the individual continues until the step is completed.

  Sequences—Performs steps in an effective or logical order for efficient use of time and energy and with an absence of (a) randomness in the ordering and/or (b) inappropriate repetition ("reordering") of steps.

  Terminates—Brings to completion single actions or single steps without perseveration, inappropriate persistence, or premature cessation.

- *Organizing space and objects*—Pertains to skills for organizing task spaces and task objects.

  Searches/locates—Looks for and locates tools and materials in a logical manner, including looking beyond the immediate environment (e.g., looking in, behind, on top of).

  Gathers—Collects needed or misplaced tools and materials, including (a) collecting located supplies into the work space and (b) collecting and replacing materials that have spilled, fallen, or been misplaced.

  Organizes—Logically positions or spatially arranges tools and materials in an orderly fashion (a) within a single work space and (b) among multiple appropriate work spaces to facilitate ease of task performance.

  Restores—(a) Puts away tools and materials in appropriate places, (b) restores immediate work space to original condition (e.g., any plastic bags to seal).

BOX A-2	PERFORMANCE SKILLS *(Continued)*

Navigates—Modifies the movement pattern of the arm, body, or wheelchair to maneuver around obstacles that are encountered in the course of moving through space such that undesirable contact with obstacles (e.g., knocking over, bumping into) is avoided (includes maneuvering objects held in the hand around obstacles).

- *Adaptation*—Relates to the ability to anticipate, correct for, and benefit by learning from the consequences of errors that arise in the course of task performance.

  Notices/responds—Responds appropriately to (a) nonverbal environmental/perceptual cues (i.e., movement, sound, smell, heat, moisture, texture, shape, consistency) that provide feedback with respect to task progression and (b) the spatial arrangement of objects to one another (e.g., aligning objects during stacking). Notices and, when indicated, makes an effective and efficient response.

  Accommodates—Modifies his or her actions or the location of objects within the work space in anticipation of or in response to problems that might arise. The client anticipates or responds to problems effectively by (a) changing the method with which he or she is performing an action sequence, (b) changing the manner in which he or she interacts with or handles tools and materials already in the work space, and (c) asking for assistance when appropriate or needed.

  Adjusts—Changes working environments in anticipation of or in response to problems that might arise. The client anticipates or responds to problems effectively by making some change (a) between working environments by moving to a new work space or bringing in or removing tools and materials from the present work space or (b) in an environmental condition (e.g., turning on or off the tap, turning up or down the temperature).

  Benefits—Anticipates and prevents undesirable circumstances or problems from recurring or persisting.

Communication/interaction skills—Refers to conveying intentions and needs and coordinating social behavior to act together with people (Forsyth and Kielhofner, 1999; Forsyth et al., 1997; Kielhofner, in press).

- *Physicality*—Pertains to using the physical body when communicating within an occupation.

  Contacts—Makes physical contact with others.

  Gazes—Uses eyes to communicate and interact with others.

(continued)

BOX A-2	PERFORMANCE SKILLS *(Continued)*

Gestures—Uses movements of the body to indicate, demonstrate, or add emphasis.

Maneuvers—Moves one's body in relation to others.

Orients—Directs one's body in relation to others and/or occupational forms.

Postures—Assumes physical positions.

- *Information exchange*—Refers to giving and receiving information within an occupation.

Articulates—Produces clear, understandable speech.

Asserts—Directly expresses desires, refusals, and requests.

Asks—Requests factual or personal information.

Engages—Initiates interactions.

Expresses—Displays affect/attitude.

Modulates—Uses volume and inflection in speech.

Shares—Gives out factual or personal information.

Speaks—Makes oneself understood through use of words, phrases, and sentences.

Sustains—Keeps up speech for appropriate duration.

- *Relations*—Relates to maintaining appropriate relationships within an occupation.

Collaborates—Coordinates action with others toward a common end goal.

Conforms—Follows implicit and explicit social norms.

Focuses—Directs conversation and behavior to ongoing social action.

Relates—Assumes a manner of acting that tries to establish a rapport with others.

Respects—Accommodates other peoples' reactions and requests.

The motor and process skills sections of this table were compiled from the following sources: Fisher (2001), Fisher and Kielhofner (1995)—updated by Fisher (2001), based on World Health Organization (2000). The Communication/interaction skills section of this table was compiled from the following sources: Forsyth and Kielhofner (1999), Forsyth et al. (1997), and Kielhofner (2002).

| **TABLE A-1** | PERFORMANCE PATTERNS |

Patterns of behavior related to daily life activities that are habitual or routine.

Habits—"Automatic behavior that is integrated into more complex patterns that enable people to function on a day-to-day basis" (Neistadt and Crepeau, 1998, p. 869). Habits can either support or interfere with performance in areas of occupation.

Type of Habit	Examples
Useful habits ■ Habits that support performance in daily life and contribute to life satisfaction. ■ Habits that support ability to follow rhythms of daily life.	■ Always put car keys in the same place so they can be found easily. ■ Brush teeth every morning to maintain good oral hygiene.
Impoverished habits ■ Habits that are not established. ■ Habits that need practice to improve.	■ Inconsistently remembering to look both ways before crossing the street.
Dominating habits ■ Habits that are so demanding they interfere with daily life. ■ Habits that satisfy a compulsive need for order	■ Inability to complete all steps of a self-care routine. ■ Repetitive self-stimulation such as type occurring in autism. ■ Use of chemical substances, resulting in addiction. ■ Neatly arranging forks on top of each other in silverware drawer.

Routines—"Occupations with established sequences" (Christiansen & Baum,1997, p.6).
Roles—"A set of behaviors that have some socially agreed on function and for which there is an accepted code of norms" (Christiansen and Baum, 1997, p. 603).

Information for the Habits section of this table was adapted from Dunn (2000).

TABLE A-2	CONTEXTS

Context (including cultural, physical, social, personal, spiritual, temporal, and virtual) refers to a variety of interrelated conditions within and surrounding the client that influence performance.

Context	Definition	Example
Physical	Customs, beliefs, activity patterns, behavior standards, and expectations accepted by the society of which the individual is a member. Includes political aspects, such as laws that affect access to resources and affirm personal rights. Also includes opportunities for education, employment, and economic support.	Ethnicity, family, attitude, beliefs, values
Physical	Nonhuman aspects of contexts. Includes the accessibility to and performance within environments having natural terrain, plants, animals, buildings, furniture, objects, tools, or devices.	Objects, built environment, natural environment, geographic terrain, sensory qualities of environment
Social	Availability and expectations of significant individuals, such as spouse, friends, and caregivers. Also includes larger social groups that are influential in establishing norms, role expectations, and social routines.	Relationships with individuals, groups, or organizations; relationships with systems (political, economic, institutional)
Personal	"Features of the individual that are not part of a health condition or health status" (WHO, 2001, p. 17). Personal context includes age, gender, socioeconomic status, and educational status.	25-year-old unemployed man with a high school diploma
Spiritual	The fundamental orientation of a person's life; that which inspires and motivates that individual.	Essence of the person, greater or higher purpose, meaning, substance
Temporal	"Location of occupational performance in time" (Neistadt and Crepeau, 1998, p. 292).	Stages of life, time of day, time of year, duration

Some of the definitions for areas of context or contexts are from the rescinded *Uniform Terminology for Occupational Therapy—Third Edition* (AOTA, 1994).

TABLE A-3	ACTIVITY DEMANDS

The aspects of an activity, including the objects, space, social demands, sequencing or timing, required actions, and required underlying body functions and body structure, needed to carry out the activity.

Definition	Examples
Objects and their properties The tools, materials, and equipment used in the process of carrying out the activity	<ul><li>Tools (scissors, dishes, shoes, volleyball)</li><li>Materials (paints, milk, lipstick)</li><li>Equipment (workbench, stove, basketball hoop)</li><li>Inherent properties (heavy, rough, sharp, colorful, loud, bitter tasting)</li></ul>
Space demands (relates to physical context) The physical environmental requirements of the activity (e.g., size, arrangement, surface, lighting, temperature, noise, humidity, ventilation)	<ul><li>Large open space outdoors required for a baseball game</li></ul>
Social demands (relates to social and cultural contexts) The social structure and demands that may be required by the activity	<ul><li>Rules of game</li><li>Expectations of other participants in activity (e.g., sharing of supplies)</li></ul>
Sequence and timing The process used to carry out the activity (specific steps, sequence, timing requirements)	<ul><li>Steps—to make tea: gather cup and tea bag, heat water, pour water into cup, etc.</li><li>Sequence—heat water before placing tea bag in water</li><li>Timing—leave tea bag to steep for 2 min</li></ul>
Required actions The usual skills that would be required by any performer to carry out the activity. Motor, process, and communication interaction skills should each be considered. The performance skills demanded by an activity will be correlated with the demands of the other activity aspects (i.e., objects, pace).	<ul><li>Gripping handlebar</li><li>Choosing a dress from the closet</li><li>Answering a question</li></ul>

(continued)

TABLE A-3 ACTIVITY DEMANDS *(Continued)*

Required body functions "The physiological functions of body systems (including psychological functions)" (WHO, 2001, p. 10) that are required to support the actions used to perform . the activity	▪ Mobility of joints ▪ Level of consciousness
Required body structures "Anatomical parts of the body such as organs, limbs, and their components [that support body function]" (WHO, 2001, p. 10) that are required to perform the activity.	▪ Number of hands ▪ Number of eyes

TABLE A-4 | CLIENT FACTORS

Those factors that reside within the client and that may affect performance in areas of occupation. Client factors include body functions and body structures. Knowledge about body functions and structures is considered when determining which functions and structures are needed to carry out an occupation/activity and how the body functions and structures may be changed as a result of engaging in an occupation/activity.

Body functions are "the physiological functions of body systems (including psychological functions)" (WHO, 2001, p. 10). Body structures are "anatomical parts of the body such as organs, limbs and their components [that support body function]" (WHO, 2001, p. 10).

Client Factor	Selected Classifications From ICF and Occupational Therapy Examples
	Body Function Categories
Mental functions (affective, cognitive, perceptual) ■ Global mental functions	■ *Consciousness functions*—level of arousal, level of consciousness. ■ *Orientation functions*—to person, place, time, self, and others. ■ *Sleep*—amount and quality of sleep. *Note:* Sleep and sleep patterns are assessed in relation to how they affect ability to effectively engage in occupations and in daily life activities. ■ *Temperament and personality functions*—conscientiousness, emotional stability, openness to experience. *Note:* These functions are assessed relative to their influence on the ability to engage in occupations and in daily life activities. ■ *Energy and drive functions*—motivation, impulse control, interests, values.

(continued)

TABLE A-4 CLIENT FACTORS (Continued)

Client Factor	Selected Classifications From ICF and Occupational Therapy Examples
	Body Function Categories
▪ Specific mental functions	▪ *Attention functions*—sustained attention, divided attention.
	▪ *Memory functions*—retrospective memory, prospective memory.
	▪ *Perceptual functions*—visuospatial perception, interpretation of sensory stimuli (tactile, visual, auditory, olfactory, gustatory).
	▪ *Thought functions*—recognition, categorization, generalization, awareness of reality, a logical/coherent thought, appropriate thought content.
	▪ *Higher-level cognitive functions*—judgment, concept formation, time management, problem solving, decision making.
	▪ *Mental functions of language*—able to receive language and express self through spoken and written or sign language. *Note:* This function is assessed relative to its influence on the ability to engage in occupations and in daily life activities.
	▪ *Calculation functions*—able to add or subtract. *Note:* These functions are assessed relative to their influence on the ability to engage in occupations and in daily life activities (e.g., making change when shopping).
	▪ *Mental functions of sequencing complex movement*—motor planning.
	▪ *Psychomotor functions*—appropriate range and regulation of motor response to psychological events.
	▪ *Emotional functions*—appropriate range and regulation of emotions, self-control.
	▪ *Experience of self and time functions*—body image, self-concept, self-esteem.
Sensory functions and pain ▪ Seeing and related functions	▪ *Seeing functions*—visual acuity, visual field functions.

(continued)

■ Hearing and vestibular functions	■ *Hearing function*—response to sound. *Note:* This function is assessed in terms of its presence or absence and its effect on engagement in everyday life activities and occupations. ■ *Vestibular function*—balance.
■ Additional sensory functions	■ *Taste function*—ability to discriminate tastes. ■ *Smell function*—ability to discriminate smells. ■ *Proprioceptive function*—kinesthesia, joint position sense. ■ *Touch functions related to temperature and other stimuli*—sensitivity to temperature, sensitivity to pressure, ability to discriminate temperature and pressure.
■ Pain	■ *Sensations of pain*—dull pain, stabbing pain.
Neuromusculoskeletal and movement-related functions ■ Functions of joints and bones	■ *Mobility of joint functions*—passive range of motion. ■ *Stability of joint functions*—postural alignment. *Note.* This refers to physiological stability of the joint related to its structural integrity compared with the motor skill of aligning the body while moving in relation to task objects. ■ *Mobility of bone functions*—frozen scapula movement of carpal bones.
■ Muscle functions	■ *Muscle power functions*—strength. ■ *Muscle tone functions*—degree of muscle tone (e.g., flaccidity, spasticity). ■ *Muscle endurance functions*—endurance.
■ Movement functions	■ *Motor reflex functions*—stretch reflex, asymmetrical tonic neck reflex. ■ *Involuntary movement reaction functions*—righting reactions, supporting reactions. ■ *Control of voluntary movement functions*—eye-hand coordination, bilateral integration, eye-foot coordination. ■ *Involuntary movement functions*—tremors, tics, motor perseveration. ■ *Gait pattern functions*—walking patterns and impairments, such as asymmetric gait, stiff gait. *(Note:* Gait patterns are assessed in relation to how they affect ability to engage in occupations and in daily life activities.)

TABLE A-4 | CLIENT FACTORS *(Continued)*

Client Factor	Selected Classifications From ICF and Occupational Therapy Examples
	Body Function Categories
Cardiovascular, hematologic, immunologic, and respiratory system function ■ Cardiovascular system function ■ Hematologic and immuno-logic system function	■ *Blood pressure functions*—hypertension, hypotension, postural hypotension. Occupational therapists and occupational therapy assistants have knowledge of these body functions and understand broadly the interaction that occurs between these functions and engagement in occupation to support participation. Some therapists may specialize in evaluating and intervening with a specific function as it is related to supporting performance and engagement in occupations and activities targeted for intervention.
■ Respiratory system function ■ Additional functions and sensations of the cardiovas-cular and respiratory systems	■ *Respiration functions*—rate, rhythm, and depth. ■ *Exercise tolerance functions*—physical endurance, aerobic capacity, stamina, and fatigability.

Voice and speech functions	Occupational therapists and occupational therapy assistants have knowledge of these body functions and understand broadly the interaction that occurs between these functions and engagement in occupation to support participation. Some therapists may specialize in evaluating and intervening with a specific function as it is related to supporting performance and engagement in occupations and activities targeted for intervention.
Digestive, metabolic, and endocrine system function ■ Metabolic system and endocrine system function ■ Digestive system function	
Genitourinary and reproductive functions ■ Urinary functions ■ Genital and reproductive functions	
Skin and related structure functions ■ Skin functions ■ Hair and nail functions	■ *Protective functions of the skin*—presence or absence of wounds, cuts, or abrasions. ■ *Repair function of the skin*—wound healing. Occupational therapists and occupational therapy assistants have knowledge of these body functions and understand broadly the interaction that occurs between these functions and engagement in occupation to support participation. Some therapists may specialize in evaluating and intervening with a specific function as it is related to supporting performance and engagement in occupations and activities targeted for intervention.

(continued)

TABLE A-4 CLIENT FACTORS *(Continued)*

Client Factor	Selected Classifications From ICF and Occupational Therapy Examples
	Body Structure Categories
■ Structure of the nervous system ■ The eye, ear, and related structures ■ Structures involved in voice and speech ■ Structures of the cardiovascular, immunologic, and respiratory systems ■ Structures related to the digestive system ■ Structures related to the genito-urinary and reproductive systems ■ Structures related to movement ■ Skin and related structures	Occupational therapists and occupational therapy assistants have knowledge of these body structures and understand broadly the interaction that occurs between these structures and engagement in occupation to support participation. Some therapists may specialize in evaluating and intervening with a specific body structure as it is related to supporting performance and engaging in occupations and activities targeted for intervention.

The reader is strongly encouraged to use International Classification of Functioning, Disability and Health (ICF) in collaboration with this table to provide for in-depth information with respect to classification in terms (inclusion and exclusion).

A Categories and classifications are adapted from the ICF (WHO, 2001).

B Categories are from the ICF (WHO, 2001).

B

Definitions and Policies for Early-Intervention Services

Reprinted from the Individuals With Disabilities Education Act, Part C. Available at:http://www.ideapractices.org. 1997.

EARLY-INTERVENTION SERVICES

Early-intervention services are developmental services that meet the following criteria:

1. Are provided under public supervision.
2. Are provided at no cost except where federal or state law provides for a system of payments by families, including a schedule of sliding fees.
3. Are designed to meet the developmental needs of an infant or toddler with a disability in any one or more of the following areas: (i) physical development, (ii) cognitive development, (iii) communication development, (iv) social or emotional development, or (v) adaptive development.
4. Meet the standards of the state in which they are provided, including the requirements of this part.
5. Include (i) family training, counseling, and home visits; (ii) special instruction; (iii) speech-language pathology and audiology services; (iv) occupational therapy; (v) physical therapy; (vi) psychological services; (vii) service coordination services; (viii) medical services only for diagnostic or evaluation

purposes; (ix) early identification, screening, and assessment services; (x) health services necessary to enable the infant or toddler to benefit from the other early intervention services; (xi) social work services; (xii) vision services; (xiii) assistive technology devices and assistive technology services; and (xiv) transportation and related costs that are necessary to enable an infant or toddler and the family to receive another service described in this paragraph.

6. Are provided by qualified personnel, including (i) special educators, (ii) speech-language pathologists and audiologists, (iii) occupational therapists, (iv) physical therapists, (v) psychologists, (vi) social workers, (vii) nurses, (viii) nutritionists, (ix) family therapists, (x) orientation and mobility specialists, and (xi) pediatricians and other physicians.

7. To the maximum extent appropriate, are provided in natural environments, including the home and community settings in which children without disabilities participate.

8. Are provided in conformity with an individual family services plan adopted in accordance with section 636.

ASSESSMENT AND PROGRAM DEVELOPMENT OF EARLY-INTERVENTION SERVICES

The individual family services plan shall be in writing and contain the following:

1. A statement of the infant's or toddler's present levels of physical development, cognitive development, communication development, social or emotional development, and adaptive development, based on objective criteria.

2. A statement of the family's resources, priorities, and concerns relating to enhancing the development of the family's infant or toddler with a disability.

3. A statement of the major outcomes expected to be achieved for the infant or toddler and the family and the criteria, procedures, and timelines used to deter-

mine the degree to which progress toward achieving the outcomes is being made and whether modifications or revisions of the outcomes or services are necessary.

4. A statement of specific early-intervention services necessary to meet the unique needs of the infant or toddler and the family, including the frequency, intensity, and method of delivering services.

5. A statement of the natural environments in which early-intervention services shall appropriately be provided, including a justification of the extent, if any, to which the services will not be provided in a natural environment.

6. The projected dates for initiation of services and the anticipated duration of the services.

7. The identification of the service coordinator from the profession most immediately relevant to the infant's or toddler's or family's needs (or who is otherwise qualified to carry out all applicable responsibilities under this part) who will be responsible for the implementation of the plan and coordination with other agencies and persons.

8. The steps to be taken to support the transition of the toddler with a disability to preschool or other appropriate services.

Definitions and Policies of the Individuals With Disabilities Education Act, Part B

Reprinted from the Individuals With Disabilities Education Act, Part B. Available at: http://www.ideapractices.org. 1997.

DEFINITIONS

Free Appropriate Public Education

Free appropriate public education is available to all children with disabilities residing in the state between ages 3 and 21 years, inclusive, including children with disabilities who have been suspended or expelled from school.

Individual Education Program

An individual education program, or an individual family services plan, that meets the federal Individuals With Disabilities Education Act requirements and is developed, reviewed, and revised for each child with a disability in accordance with the law.

Least Restrictive Environment

In general, to the maximum extent appropriate, children with disabilities, including children in public or private institutions or other care facilities, are educated with children who are not disabled. Special classes, separate schooling, or other removal of children with disabilities from the regular educational environment occurs only when the nature or severity of the disability of a child is such that education in regular classes with the use of supplementary aids and services cannot be achieved satisfactorily.

POLICIES

Conducting Initial Evaluations

In general, the state educational agency, other state agency, or local educational agency shall conduct a full and individual initial evaluation before the initial provision of special education and related services to a child with a disability. Such initial evaluation shall consist of procedures: (1) to determine whether a child is a child with a disability and (2) to determine the educational needs of such child.

Reevaluations

A local educational agency shall ensure that a reevaluation of each child with a disability is conducted if conditions warrant a reevaluation or if the child's parent or teacher requests a reevaluation, but at least once every 3 years.

Evaluation Procedures

The local educational agency shall provide notice to the parents of a child with a disability in accordance with the law that describes any evaluation procedures such agency proposes to conduct. In conducting the evaluation, the local educational agency shall (1) use a variety of assessment tools and strategies to gather relevant functional and developmental information, including information provided by the parent, that may assist in determining whether the child is a child with a disability and the content of the child's individual education program, including information related to enabling the child to be involved in and progress in the general curriculum or, for preschool children, to participate in appropriate activities; (2) not use any single procedure as the sole criterion for determining whether a child is a child with a disability or for determining an appropriate educational program for the child; and (3) use technically sound instruments that may assess the relative contribution of cognitive and behavioral factors in addition to physical or developmental factors.

In addition, each local educational agency shall ensure that (1) tests and other evaluation materials used to assess a child are selected and administered so as not to be discriminatory on a racial or cultural basis; (2) tests and other evaluation materials are provided and administered in the child's native language or other mode of communication, unless it is clearly not feasible to do so; (3) any standardized tests that are given to the child have been validated for the specific purpose for which they are used, are administered by trained and knowledgeable personnel, and are administered in accordance with any instructions provided by the producer of such tests; and (4) the child is assessed in all areas of suspected disability and assessment tools and strategies that provide relevant information that directly assists persons in determining the educational needs of the child are provided.

Additional Requirements for Evaluation and Reevaluations

As part of an initial evaluation (if appropriate) and as part of any reevaluation under the individual education program team described in subsection and other qualified professionals, as appropriate, shall:

1. Review existing evaluation data on the child, including evaluations and information provided by the parents of the child, current classroom-based assessments and observations, and teacher and related service provider observation.
2. On the basis of that review, and input from the child's parents, identify what additional data, if any, are needed to determine whether the child has a partic-

ular category of disability, or, in case of a reevaluation of a child, whether the child continues to have such a disability. Data are also needed to identify the present levels of performance and the educational needs of the child, whether the child needs special education and related services, or, in the case of a reevaluation of a child, whether the child continues to need special education and related services, and whether any additions or modifications to the special education and related services are needed to enable the child to meet the measurable annual goals set out in the individual education program of the child and to participate, as appropriate, in the general curriculum.

Individual Education Programs

The term *individual education program* means a written statement for each child with a disability that is developed, reviewed, and revised in accordance with this section and that includes the following:

1. A statement of the child's present levels of educational performance, including how the child's disability affects the child's involvement and progress in the general curriculum, or, for preschool children, as appropriate, how the disability affects the child's participation in appropriate activities.
2. A statement of measurable annual goals, including benchmarks or short-term objectives related to meeting the child's needs that result from the child's disability to enable the child to be involved in and progress in the general curriculum and to meeting each of the child's other educational needs that result from the child's disability.
3. A statement of the special education and related services and supplementary aids and services to be provided to the child or on behalf of the child.
4. A statement of the program modifications or support for school personnel that will be provided for the child (1) to advance appropriately toward attaining the annual goals, to be involved and

progress in the general curriculum, and to participate in extracurricular and other nonacademic activities and (2) to be educated and participate with other children with disabilities and nondisabled children in the activities described in this paragraph.

5. An explanation of the extent, if any, to which the child will not participate with nondisabled children in regular class activities.

6. A statement of any individual modifications in the administration of state- or district-wide assessments of student achievement that are needed for the child to participate in such assessment.

7. If the individual education program team determines that the child will not participate in a particular state- or district-wide assessment of student achievement (or part of such an assessment), a statement of why that assessment is not appropriate for the child and how the child will be assessed.

8. The projected date for the beginning of the special education and related services and modifications described and the anticipated frequency, location, and duration of those services and modifications.

9. Beginning at age 14 years, and updated annually, a statement of the transition service needs of the child under the applicable components of the child's individual education program that focuses on the child's courses of study (such as participation in advanced-placement courses or a vocational education program).

10. Beginning at age 16 years (or younger as determined to be appropriate by the individual education program team), a statement of needed transition services for the child, including, when appropriate, a statement of the interagency responsibilities or any needed linkages.

Education Services Provided Through Section 504 of the Rehabilitation Act of 1973

Information in this section is from the following Web sites: www.reedmartin.com/section504.html; www.ed.gov/offices /OCR.

DESCRIPTION OF SECTION 504

"Section 504" was passed by Congress as the final section of the Rehabilitation Act of 1973, which was Public Law 93-112. It is placed in the United States Code (USC) at Title 29 USC Section 794. If you read judicial decisions on special education, the judge might refer to it as "Section 504" or as "Section 794." Section 504 states that "no qualified individual with a disability in the United States shall be excluded from, denied the benefits of, or be subjected to discrimination under" any *program or activity* that either receives federal financial assistance or is conducted by any executive agency or the United States Postal Service. Each federal agency has its own set of section 504 regulations that apply to its own programs. Agencies that provide federal financial assistance also have section 504 regulations covering entities that receive federal aid. Requirements common to these regulations include reasonable accommodation for employees with disabilities, program accessibility, effective communication with people who have hearing or vision disabilities, and accessible new construction and alterations. Each agency is responsible for enforcing its own regulations. Section 504 may also be enforced through private lawsuits. It is not necessary to file a complaint with a federal agency or to receive a "right-to-sue" letter before going to court.

For the purposes of this section, the term *program or activity* means all of the operations of various agencies and organizations or other instrumentality of a state or local government, including a college, university, or other postsecondary institution, or a public system of higher education; or a local educational agency as defined in section 14101 of the Elementary and Secondary Education Act of 1965, system of vocational education, or other school system.

EVALUATION AND PLACEMENT

Preplacement Evaluation

A recipient that operates a public elementary or secondary education program shall conduct an evaluation, in accordance with the requirements of the evaluation procedures in this section, of any person who, because of handicap, needs or is believed to need special education or related services before taking any action with respect to the initial placement of the person in a regular or special education program and any subsequent significant change in placement.

Evaluation Procedures

A recipient to which this subpart applies shall establish standards and procedures for the evaluation and placement of persons who, because of handicap, need or are believed to need special education or related services that ensure that (1) tests and other evaluation materials have been validated for the specific purpose for which they are used and are administered by trained personnel in conformance with the instructions provided by their producer; (2) tests and other evaluation materials include those tailored to assess specific areas of educational need and not merely those designed to provide a single general intelligence quotient; and (3) tests are selected and administered so as to best ensure that, when a test is administered to a student with impaired sensory, manual, or speaking skills, the test results accurately reflect the student's aptitude or achievement level or whatever other factor the test purports to measure, rather than reflecting the student's impaired sensory, manual, or speaking skills (except where those skills are the factors that the test purports to measure).

Placement Procedures

In interpreting evaluation data and in making placement decisions, a recipient shall (1) draw on information from a variety of sources, including aptitude and achievement tests, teacher recommendations, physical condition, social or cultural background, and adaptive behavior; (2) establish procedures to ensure that information obtained from all such sources is documented and carefully considered; (3) ensure that the placement decision is made by a group of persons, including persons knowledgeable about the child, the meaning of the evaluation data, and the placement options; and (4) ensure that the placement decision is made in conformity with 104.34.

Reevaluation

A recipient to whom this section applies shall establish procedures, in accordance with paragraph (b) of this section, for periodic reevaluation of students who have been provided special education and related services. A reevaluation procedure consistent with the Education for the Handicapped Act is one means of meeting this requirement.

Definitions From the International Classification of Functioning, Disability, and Health (ICF, World Health Organization) and the American Occupational Therapy Association (AOTA) Uniform Terminology

ICF DEFINITIONS IN THE CONTEXT OF HEALTH

(From the World Health Organization Web site. Available at: http://www.who.int/icf.)

Body functions are the physiologic functions of body systems (including psychological functions).

Body structures are the anatomic parts of the body, such as organs, limbs, and their components.

Impairments are problems in body function or structure, such as a significant deviation or loss.

Activity is the execution of a task or action by an individual.

Participation is involvement in a life situation.

Activity limitations are difficulties an individual may have in executing activities.

Participation restrictions are problems an individual may experience in involvement in life situations.

Environmental factors make up the physical, social, and attitudinal environment in which people live and conduct their lives.

AOTA'S UNIFORM TERMINOLOGY

Figure E-1 is taken from an official document of the AOTA. This document was intended to provide a generic outline of the domain of concern for occupational therapy and to provide common terminology for the profession. This terminology was incorporated into the more recent AOTA Occupational Therapy Practice Framework.

I. Performance Areas

A. Activities of Daily Living
1. Grooming
2. Oral Hygiene
3. Bathing/Showering
4. Toilet Hygiene
5. Personal Device Care
6. Dressing
7. Feeding and Eating
8. Medication Routine
9. Health Maintenance
10. Socialization
11. Functional Communication
12. Functional Mobility
13. Community Mobility
14. Emergency Response
15. Sexual Expression
B. Work and Productive Activities
  1. Home Management
    a. Clothing Care

    b. Cleaning
    c. Meal Preparation/Cleanup
    d. Shopping
    e. Money Management
    f. Household Maintenance
    g. Safety Procedures
  2. Care of Others
  3. Educational Activities
  4. Vocational Activities
    a. Vocational Exploration
    b. Job Acquisition
    c. Work or Job Performance
    d. Retirement Planning
    e. Volunteer Participation
C. Play or Leisure Activities
  1. Play or Leisure Exploration
  2. Play or Leisure Performance

(continued)

Figure E-1. Uniform Terminology for Occupational Therapy, Third Edition Outline. (Reprinted with permission from American Occupational Therapy Association. Uniform Terminology for Occupational Therapy, Third Edition. *Am J Occup Ther* 1994;48:1047–1054.)

Figure E-1. *(Continued)*

II. Performance Components

A. Sensorimotor Component
  1. Sensory
    a. Sensory Awareness
    b. Sensory Processing
      (1) Tactile
      (2) Proprioceptive
      (3) Vestibular
      (4) Visual
      (5) Auditory
      (6) Gustatory
      (7) Olfactory
    c. Perceptual Processing
      (1) Stereognosis
      (2) Kinesthesia
      (3) Pain Response
      (4) Body Scheme
      (5) Right-Left
        Discrimination
      (6) Form Constancy
      (7) Position in Space
      (8) Visual-Closure
      (9) Figure Ground
      (10) Depth Perception
      (11) Spatial Relations
      (12) Topographical
        Orientation
  2. Neuromusculoskeletal
    a. Reflex
    b. Range of Motion
    c. Muscle Tone
    d. Strength
    e. Endurance
    f. Postural Control
    g. Postural Alignment
    h. Soft Tissue Integrity
  3. Motor
    a. Gross Coordination
    b. Crossing the Midline
    c. Literality
    d. Bilateral Integration
    e. Motor Control
    f. Praxis
    g. Fine Coordination/
      Dexterity
      h. Visual-Motor
        Integration
      i. Oral-Motor Control
B. Cognitive Integration and
  Cognitive Components
  1. Level of Arousal
  2. Orientation
  3. Recognition
  4. Attention Span
  5. Initiation of Activity
  6. Termination of Activity
  7. Memory
  8. Sequencing
  9. Categorization
  10. Concept Formation
  11. Spatial Operations
  12. Problem Solving
  13. Learning
  14. Generalization
C. Psychosocial Skills and
  Psychological Components
  1. Psychological
    a. Values
    b. Interests
    c. Self-Concept
  2. Social
    a. Role Performance
    b. Social Conduct
    c. Interpersonal Skills
    d. Self-Expression
  3. Self-Management
    a. Coping Skills
    b. Time Management
    c. Self-Control

III. Performance Contexts

A. Temporal Aspects
  1. Chronological
  2. Developmental
  3. Life Cycle
  4. Disability Status
B. Environment
  1. Physical
  2. Social
  3. Cultural

RELATIONSHIP OF THE AOTA PRACTICE FRAMEWORK TO THE RESCINDED UNIFORM TERMINOLOGY III AND THE ICF

(Reprinted with permission from the American Occupational Therapy Association, 2002.) Available at: http://www.aota.org. 2002, and the *American Journal of Occupational Therapy*.

The Practice Framework updates, revises, and incorporates the primary elements (performance areas, performance components, and performance contexts) outlined in the rescinded Uniform Terminology III. In some cases, the names of these elements were updated to reflect shifts in thinking and to create more obvious links with terminology outside of the profession. Feedback from reviews indicated that the use of occupational therapy terminology often made it more difficult for others to understand what occupational therapy contributes. The ICF language was also seen as important to incorporate. Table E-1 shows how terminology has evolved by comparing terminology used in the Practice Framework, the rescinded Uniform Terminology III, and the ICF documents.

TABLE E-1

Occupational Therapy Practice Framework: Domain and Process	Rescinded UT-III[a]	ICF[b]
		Interactions and relationships, major life areas, community, social and civic life. Activities and Participation examples from *ICF* overlap Areas of Occupation, Performance Skills, and Performance Patterns in the *Framework*.
Context or **Contexts**—refers to a variety of inter-related conditions within and surrounding the client that influence performance. Context includes cultural, physical, social, personal, spiritual, temporal, and virtual contexts.	**Performance Contexts** (p. 1054)— ■ *Temporal Aspects* (chronological, developmental, life cycle, disability status) ■ *Environment* (physical, social, cultural)	**Contextual Factors**—"represent the complete background of an individual's life and living. They include environmental factors and personal factors that may have an effect on the individual with a health condition and the individual's health and health-related states" (p. 16). ■ *Environmental factors*—"make up the physical, social and attitudinal environment in which people live and conduct their lives. The factors are external to individuals . . ." (p. 16). ■ *Personal factors*—"the particular background of an individual's life and living . . ." (p. 17) (e.g., gender, race, lifestyle, habits, social background, education, profession). Personal factors are not classified in *ICF* because they are not part of a health condition or health state, though they are recognized as having an effect on outcomes.

(continued)

TABLE E-1 (Continued)

Occupational Therapy Practice Framework: Domain and Process	Rescinded UT-III[a]	ICF[b]
Activity Demands—the aspects of an activity, which include the objects, space, social demands, sequencing or timing, required actions, and required underlying body functions and body structures needed to carry out the activity.	Not addressed	Not addressed
Client Factors—those factors that reside within the client that may affect performance in areas of occupation. Client factors include the following: ■ *Body functions*—"the physiological functions of body systems (including psychological functions)" (WHO, 2001, p. 10). ■ *Body Structures*—"anatomical parts of the body such as organs, limbs and their components [that support body function]" (WHO, 2001, p. 10).	**Performance Components** sensorimotor components, cognitive interaction and cognitive components, as well as psychosocial skills and psychological components. These components consist of some performance skills and some client factors as presented in the *Framework* (pp.. 1052–1054).	■ *Body Functions*—"the physiological functions of body systems (including psychological functions)" (p. 10). ■ *Body Structures*—"anatomical parts of the body such as organs, limbs and their components [that support body function]" (p. 10).
Outcomes—important dimensions of health attributed to interventions, including ability to function, health perceptions, and satisfaction with care (adapted from Request for Planning Ideas, 2001).	Not addressed	Not addressed

[a]American Occupational Therapy Association (1994).
[b]World Health Organization (2001).
Adapted and reprinted from The American Occupational Therapy Association. (2002). *Occupational Therapy Practice Framework*. Available at:http://www.AOTA.org

American Occupational Therapy Association Code of Ethics

The text in this appendix has been reprinted with permission from the American Occupational Therapy Association. American Occupational Therapy Code of Ethics. Available at: http://www.aota.org. 2002.

PREAMBLE

The American Occupational Therapy Association's (AOTA's) Code of Ethics is a public statement of the common set of values and principles used to promote and maintain high standards of behavior in occupational therapy. The AOTA and its members are committed to furthering the ability of individuals, groups, and systems to function within their total environment. To this end, occupational therapy personnel (including all staff and personnel who work and assist in providing occupational therapy services, e.g., aides, orderlies, secretaries, and technicians) have a responsibility to provide services to recipients in any stage of health and illness who are individuals, research participants, institutions and businesses, other professionals and colleagues, and students and to the general public.

The Occupational Therapy Code of Ethics is a set of principles that applies to occupational therapy personnel at all levels. These principles to which occupational therapists and occupational therapy assistants aspire are part of a lifelong effort to act in an ethical manner. The various roles of practitioner (occupational therapist and occupational therapy assistant), educator, fieldwork educator, clinical supervisor, manager, administrator, consultant, fieldwork coordinator, faculty program director, researcher/scholar, private practice owner, entrepreneur, and student are assumed.

Any action in violation of the spirit and purpose of this Code shall be considered unethical. To ensure compliance with the Code, the Commission on Standards and Ethics establishes and maintains the enforcement procedures.

Acceptance of membership in the AOTA commits members to adherence to the Code of Ethics and its enforcement procedures. The Code of Ethics, Core Values, and Attitudes of Occupational Therapy Practice (AOTA, 1993), and the Guidelines to the Occupational Therapy Code of Ethics (AOTA, 1998) are aspirational documents designed to be used together to guide occupational therapy personnel.

PRINCIPLE 1

Occupational therapy personnel shall demonstrate a concern for the well-being of the recipients of their services. (beneficence)

A. Occupational therapy personnel shall provide services in a fair and equitable manner. They shall recognize and appreciate the cultural components of economics, geography, race, ethnicity, religious and political factors, marital status, sexual orientation, and disability of all recipients of their services.

B. Occupational therapy practitioners shall strive to ensure that fees are fair and reasonable and commensurate with services performed. When occupational therapy practitioners set fees, they shall set fees considering institutional, local, state, and federal requirements and with due regard for the service recipient's ability to pay.

C. Occupational therapy personnel shall make every effort to advocate for recipients to obtain needed services through available means.

PRINCIPLE 2

Occupational therapy personnel shall take reasonable precautions to avoid imposing or inflicting harm on the recipient of services or to his or her property. (nonmaleficence)

A. Occupational therapy personnel shall maintain relationships that do not exploit the recipient of services sexually, physically, emotionally, financially, socially, or in any other manner.

B. Occupational therapy practitioners shall avoid relationships or activities that interfere with professional judgment and objectivity.

PRINCIPLE 3

Occupational therapy personnel shall respect the recipients and/or their surrogate(s) as well as the recipient's rights. (autonomy, privacy, confidentiality)

A. Occupational therapy practitioners shall collaborate with service recipients or their surrogate(s) in setting goals and priorities throughout the intervention process.

B. Occupational therapy practitioners shall fully inform the service recipients of the nature, risks, and potential outcomes of any interventions.

C. Occupational therapy practitioners shall obtain informed consent from participants involved in research activities and indicate that they have fully informed and advised the participants of potential risks and outcomes. Occupational therapy practitioners shall endeavor to ensure that the participant(s) comprehend these risks and outcomes.

D. Occupational therapy personnel shall respect the individual's right to refuse professional services or involvement in research or educational activities.

E. Occupational therapy personnel shall protect all privileged confidential forms of written, verbal, and electronic communication gained from educational, practice, research, and investigational activities unless otherwise mandated by local, state, or federal regulations.

PRINCIPLE 4

Occupational therapy personnel shall achieve and continually maintain high standards of competence. (duties)

A. Occupational therapy practitioners shall hold the appropriate national and state credentials for the services they provide.

B. Occupational therapy practitioners shall use procedures that conform to the standards of practice and other appropriate AOTA documents relevant to practice.

C. Occupational therapy practitioners shall take responsibility for maintaining and documenting competence by participating in professional development and educational activities.

D. Occupational therapy practitioners shall critically examine and keep current with emerging knowledge relevant to their practice so they may perform their duties on the basis of accurate information.

E. Occupational therapy practitioners shall protect service recipients by ensuring that duties assumed by or assigned to other occupational therapy personnel match credentials, qualifications, experience, and scope of practice.

F. Occupational therapy practitioners shall provide appropriate supervision to individuals for whom the practitioners have supervisory responsibility in accordance with Association policies; local, state and federal laws; and institutional values.

G. Occupational therapy practitioners shall refer to or consult with other service providers whenever such a referral or consultation would be helpful to the care of the recipient of service. The referral or consultation process should be done in collaboration with the recipient of service.

PRINCIPLE 5

Occupational therapy personnel shall comply with laws and Association policies guiding the profession of occupational therapy. (justice)

A. Occupational therapy personnel shall familiarize themselves with and seek to understand and abide by applicable Association policies; local, state, and federal laws; and institutional rules.

B. Occupational therapy practitioners shall remain abreast of revisions in those laws and Association policies that apply to the profession of occupational therapy and shall inform employers, employees, and colleagues of those changes.

C. Occupational therapy practitioners shall require those they supervise in occupational therapy-related activities to adhere to the Code of Ethics.

D. Occupational therapy practitioners shall take reasonable steps to ensure that employers are aware of occupational therapy's ethical obligations, as set forth in this Code of Ethics, and of the implications of those obligations for occupational therapy practice, education, and research.

E. Occupational therapy practitioners shall record and report in an accurate and timely manner all information related to professional activities.

PRINCIPLE 6

Occupational therapy personnel shall provide accurate information about occupational therapy services. (veracity)

A. Occupational therapy personnel shall accurately represent their credentials, qualifications, education, experience, training, and competence. This is of particular importance for those to whom occupational therapy personnel provide their services or with whom occupational therapy practitioners have a professional relationship.

B. Occupational therapy personnel shall disclose any professional, personal, financial, business, or volunteer affiliations that may pose a conflict of interest to those with whom they may establish a professional, contractual, or other working relationship.

C. Occupational therapy personnel shall refrain from using or participating in the use of any form of communication that contains false, fraudulent, deceptive, or unfair statements or claims.

D. Occupational therapy practitioners shall accept the responsibility for their professional actions that reduce the public's trust in occupational therapy services and those that perform those services.

PRINCIPLE 7

Occupational therapy personnel shall treat colleagues and other professionals with fairness, discretion, and integrity. (fidelity)

A. Occupational therapy personnel shall preserve, respect, and safeguard confidential information about colleagues and staff, unless otherwise mandated by national, state, or local laws.

B. Occupational therapy practitioners shall accurately represent the qualifications, views, contributions, and findings of colleagues.

C. Occupational therapy personnel shall take adequate measures to discourage, prevent, expose, and correct any breaches of the Code of Ethics and report any breaches of the Code of Ethics to the appropriate authority.

D. Occupational therapy personnel shall familiarize themselves with established policies and procedures for handling concerns about this Code of Ethics, including familiarity with national, state, local, district, and territorial procedures for handling ethics complaints. These include policies and procedures created by the AOTA, licensing and regulatory bodies, employers, agencies, certification boards, and other organizations that have jurisdiction over occupational therapy practice.

References

American Occupational Therapy Association. Core values and attitudes of occupational therapy practice. *Am J Occup Ther* 1993;47:1085-1086.

American Occupational Therapy Association. Guidelines to the occupational therapy code of ethics. *Am J Occup Ther* 1998;52:881-884.

Authors The Commission on Standards and Ethics (SEC):

April 2000 Adopted by the Representative Assembly 2000 M15

Note: This document replaces the 1994 document, Occupational Therapy Code of Ethics (*Am J Occup Ther* 1994;48:1037-1038). Prepared 4/7/2000

INDEX

Page numbers in *italics* indicate figures. Page numbers followed by "t" indicate tables.